DATE DUE			

sing:
tation

Forensic Mental Health Nursing: Policy, Strategy and Implementation

PAUL TARBUCK
Director – Forensic and High Dependency Services
Mental Health Services of Salford NHS Trust

BARRY TOPPING-MORRIS
Head of Forensic Nursing
South Wales Forensic Psychiatric Services

PHILIP BURNARD
Professor and Vice Dean, School of Nursing Studies,
University of Wales College of Medicine

W

WHURR PUBLISHERS
LONDON

© 1999 Whurr Publishers
First published 1999 by
Whurr Publishers Ltd
19b Compton Terrace, London N1 2UN, England

British Library Cataloguing in Publication Data
A catalogue record for this book is available from the British
Library.

ISBN: 1 86156 128 8

Printed and bound in the UK by Athenaeum Press Ltd,
Gateshead, Tyne & Wear

Contents

Contributors

Colin Beacock Colin has extensive experience in management and educational roles in learning disability nursing and high-security nursing care. He was responsible for leading Rampton Hospital into its successful relationship with Sheffield Hallam University. Colin, along with a small group of learning disability nurses from the UK, did much to support colleagues in Eastern Europe, particularly Romania, after the fall of the Berlin Wall. He is currently an officer of the Royal College of Nursing of the United Kingdom (this chapter being written prior to his taking up this appointment).

Philip Burnard Philip Burnard is a Professor at the University of Wales College of Medicine School of Nursing and has a background in nursing, within which he has extensively researched and published. He has worked closely with the South Wales Forensic Psychiatric Services in terms of describing standards of care and in staff development.

Stephen Burrow Stephen's forensic nursing career has included research, senior nurse management and tutorial, lecturing and advisory positions in medium secure units, Special Hospitals and prison service health care. During this time, he was programme leader to the diploma in forensic mental health nursing with the University of the South Bank. Stephen has contributed regularly to professional discourse on the evolving forensic mental nurse via professional publications, and he now sits on two professional editorial boards. He is currently a forensic nurse lecturer/practitioner with a medium secure unit within the South London and Maudsley NHS Trust and holds an honorary lectureship with the Institute of Psychiatry.

Chris Chaloner Chris is a Senior Lecturer in the School of Health, University of Greenwich, London, where he specialises in Forensic Mental Health and Ethics. Chris has worked within both high and medium secure forensic services and has a particular interest in the ethical aspects of health care. He formerly worked as a Lecturer/Practitioner in Forensic Mental Health Nursing at Pathfinder NHS Trust and St. George's Hospital Medical School, London.

Yvonne Eaton From an NHS Technical Instructor career, Yvonne joined the Care and Responsibility training team at Ashworth Hospital in 1991. She was involved in developing more sensitive approaches to control and restraint training and is renowned for challenging discriminatory and 'macho' approaches to relating to assaultive patients, as well as for her work in challenging sexist attitudes in the work place. She has also helped to develop the commercially available Ashworth C&R open learning materials. Additionally, Yvonne coordinates the operational emergency response teams as the need arises at Ashworth Hospital.

Kevin Gournay Kevin is Professor of Nursing at the Institute of Psychiatry in London. He has a background in nursing and psychology, and remains a member of the British Psychological Society whilst being active in leading change in the profession of mental health nursing at national level via the Royal College of Nursing and other influential bodies. Kevin is a tireless figure in promoting the advancing and specialist role of the nurse, particularly in relation to the introduction of evidence-based practices using psychosocial and cognitive therapeutic approaches. He is extensively published and has many research and academic interests, which have led him to become well known to nurses working within medium and high secure care environments.

Frank Hanily Frank is presently the manager of an innovative Primary Mental Health Service in the Ribble Valley, East Lancashire and an Associate Consultant with the Centre for Mental Health Services Development, King's College London. He is qualified as a Mental Health Nurse, with a Degree in Law and a MSc in Research Methodology. He has a particular interest in social policy and service development. He is also a practising community mental health nurse and an active member of the RCN mental health nursing forum.

Gina Hillis Gina is known for her uncompromising approach to setting high standards within forensic services at the Reaside Clinic and is associated with groundbreaking community forensic services developments in the city of Birmingham. Latterly, Gina has been a leading figure in educational developments related to sharing good practices in community forensic mental health care, but she is careful to maintain her clinical profile.

John Kilshaw John trained at Rainhill and Whiston Hospitals, qualifying from them in 1972 and 1974 respectively. Appointed charge nurse at Mersey Region Interim Secure Unit in 1976, he then became Senior Clinical Nurse at the Scott Clinic. During his time with the forensic service, John has been a member of numerous working groups, including the planning team for the ENB 960 course and the diploma in Forensic Care and Management at Ashworth. He is a founder member of the Forensic Nurses Association and is currently Manager, Severe and Enduring Mental Illness Services at St Helens and Knowsley Hospital Trust.

Connor Kinsella Connor is currently working as a freelance trainer. He has extensive experience within forensic mental health services including positions both as a Ward Manager in a medium secure unit and as a Forensic Community Mental Health Nurse.

Neil Kitchiner Neil has experienced forensic care within Milton Keynes MSU and the Caswell Clinic, and is now practising as a Clinical Nurse Specialist within prison health care. He has extensive experience of developing court diversion schemes and now concentrates his considerable skill and knowledge in the domain of cognitive behavioural nurse psychotherapy. Neil is much travelled and occasionally published.

Joe McAuliffe Joe, a nurse, became an Instructor of Control and Restraint at Ashworth Hospital and helped to develop the Ashworth variant of C&R known as Care and Responsibility. He has wide experience of training colleagues in C&R usage throughout the UK in both the NHS and independant sectors. Joe has worked in the independant sector since 1997 and contiues to train others on a freelance basis.

Michael McCourt Michael has worked in forensic mental health services since 1988, when he commenced work as a staff nurse at Newton Lodge RSU in Yorkshire. In 1990, he moved to North Wales as a charge nurse to join a team developing new inpatient and community forensic services. He then worked in Lambeth as a team leader in forensic community services. His work since 1997 has included managing and developing services at the Cane Hill MSU. Michael is now the service lead on the Trusts Commissioning team to develop forensic services in the Borough of Lambeth.

'Harry' 'Harry' would like to thank those who have contributed to more humane treatments of their fellow men and women in secure hospitals. He is grateful to the people he knew (patients and staff) who were positive and supportive of him, and thereby helped his healing process.

David Mercer Is a lecturer in the Department of Nursing at the University of Liverpool. His career spans mental health practice, research and education, with a particular focus on the care and management of mentally disordered offenders. He previously worked in high security psychiatric services as a ward based nurse, and later as a lecturer practitioner. Current research combines clinical interest in therapeutic interventions for sexually violent men with a critical analysis of medicalised deviance and psychiatric discourse. He regularly contributes to peer reviewed journals, and has co-authored three books.

John Parry John has been the Senior Nurse Manager at the Scott Clinic medium secure unit on Merseyside since its inception. He is a senior member of the forensic mental health nursing fraternity and has done much to champion the cause of the patient, and the nurse, over 30 years of NHS service. John has been involved in a variety of national and regional innovative strategies over the years and is currently giving advice to the Regional Specialist Mental Health Commissioning Agency in the North West.

David Robinson David is Professor of Forensic Nursing at the University of Sheffield. He is a prolific researcher and publisher who has done much to further the development of enhanced standards of care at Rampton Hospital, assisting many others in describing various aspects of the enhanced role of the nurse. David has been in the forefront of utilising information technology in clinical practice and has led the development of the International Forensic Psychiatric Database which is linked with York University.

Paul Rogers Paul, a clinician, was the first nurse to work in forensic mental health with the ENB 650 qualification. He has published internationally on cognitive behavioural interventions applied in nursing and has recently attracted international interest for his work with offenders displaying post-traumatic stress disorder as a consequence of their own offending. Paul is on the Editorial Board of the journal *Mental Health Practice* and is an external reviewer for the Health Advisory Service.

Mick Ruane Mick has wide experience of nursing in a variety of NHS settings, including Park Lane Hospital, later to become known as Ashworth. Mick assisted in the development of care and responsibility training at Ashworth and is now the Control and Restraint Training Co-ordinator for Manchester Royal Hospitals NHS Trust.

David Sallah David is in the final stages of his doctoral studies and is working in independent practice as a clinician and management consultant. He has wide experience of many medium- and high-security environments in England and Wales, and is most associated with the Reaside Clinic medium secure service in Birmingham, which has acquired an international reputation in part thanks to David's endeavours. He has also worked at the Department of Health, where he co-ordinated work on the publication of the forensic mental health nursing response to the *Vision for Nursing, Midwifery and Health Visiting*. As the Editor of *Psychiatric Care*, David has done much to encourage the growth of forensic mental health nursing by encouraging many to take their first steps in publishing.

Chris Skelly Chris has extensive experience of clinical and managerial working in medium and high secure care environments, at both the Scott Clinic medium secure unit and Ashworth Hospital. Chris was one of the first group of Ward Managers who were charged with changing the culture of care at Ashworth Hospital after the first public inquiry. Chris also occasionally appears in print.

Paul Tarbuck Paul is currently the Director of the Forensic and High Dependency Services at the Mental Health Services of Salford NHS Trust. Previously, he worked for many years in an educational role at Ashworth Hospital, where the team achieved many firsts, including the first ENB 770 course and Diploma in Forensic Care. Paul has worked in many areas of England and in the Middle East, in both general and mental health nursing, as a clinician, educator and manager. He is currently giving advice to the Regional Specialist Mental Health Commissioning Agency in the North West. His work is occasionally published.

Bill Thorpe Bill is the senior Instructor of Care and Responsibility at Ashworth Hospital on Merseyside and has led the development of techniques designed to reduce physical interventions to an absolute minimum within an ethicolegal framework. Bill has worked throughout the UK and abroad, and also assists with emergency response teamworking at Ashworth.

Marie Toman Marie has extensive experience of clinical and educational working in the NHS and is currently Nurse Tutor at the Caswell Clinic medium secure services in Wales. Marie has instigated educational innovations in general psychiatric care, particularly in forensic mental health nursing. Marie occasionally appears in print and is firmly anchored in person-centred practices.

Barry Topping-Morris Barry is Head of Forensic Nursing at the Caswell Clinic, Bridgend and forensic nurse advisor to the Chief Nursing Officer at the Welsh Office, with experience at the Scott Clinic, Reaside and now Caswell Clinic MSU. He is renowned throughout the UK for his innovative approaches to care and for his tireless championing of the service user's view. The services that he manages are often quoted as examples of the best practices in medium secure care. Barry occasionally appears in print.

Preface

For most of this century, the profession of nursing within secure environments has been dormant and ignored, shut away in the depths of the prisons and veiled in secrecy within the Special Hospitals (which were, until 1989, cloaked by the Official Secrets Act). However, in the past 20 years, a specialist branch of psychiatric nursing has emerged in many parts of the UK – that of forensic nursing. Akin to other branches of psychiatric nursing, forensic nurses have chosen to adopt the title of mental health nurses. This reflects the desire to offer health-focused and holistic approaches (rather than merely pathogenic or single systems approaches) to caring. Thus, the 'new' professionals refer to themselves as forensic mental health nurses. A group of forensic mental health nurses are working in the community and are in the vanguard of changing approaches to service provision. These practititoners choose to call themselves forensic community mental health nurses.

Although forensic nurses have existed in the prisons and Special Hospitals for generations, a clear identity is only now emerging around a common understanding of the role of the forensic mental health nurse. Diverse but interrelated factors have given impetus to this change. These include:

- community-focused health and social policy, leading to the reduction of long-stay residential psychiatric facilities, which increases pressure on the remaining services and generates greater community workloads;
- the recognition of forensic psychiatry as a medical specialism;
- the growth of the psychiatric medium secure and high-dependency (low secure) care sectors, which have injected forensic care environments with energy and enthusiasm;

- the growing orientation of both the high-security hospitals and the prison health care services towards mainstream health care ethics and practices;
- the raised expectations of the public to receive timely, specialist care, available locally and on demand;
- effective politicisation of the psychiatric agenda by pressure groups and service user representative groups;
- a growing interest in mentally disordered offenders arising from the press and communication media and fuelled by a growing catalogue of failures of care in the community (some of which have led to some terrible tragedies involving mentally disordered individuals).

The first textbook related to the forensic nursing field, published in 1992, was entitled *Aspects of Forensic Psychiatric Nursing* (edited by P. Morrison and P. Burnard and published by Avebury in Aylesbury). Prior to this book, relatively few nurses working in the forensic psychiatric sector had committed their experiences and thoughts to print. Since publication of this book, however, forensic mental health nurses have made meaningful and sustained contributions to the professional literature, and forensic nursing academics are emerging to take some of the newly established Chairs in mental health nursing. There is a tangible sense that forensic nursing has arrived and is accepted by other forensic disciplines.

The willingness of forensic mental health nurses to share their practices (and their dilemmas) nearly did not occur. In the 1980s, the emerging specialty was dominated by disputes between the old (Special Hospitals) and the new (medium secure services), each viewing the other suspiciously, believing that the ideology associated with the other would 'contaminate' them. These 'birth pains' were probably inevitable as no clear definitions of 'high' and 'medium' secure care existed (and arguably still do not) and as the central dilemma of the role of the forensic mental health nurse – as carer or custodian – had still not been articulated, questioned or subjected to new paradigms. However, the impetus of English and Welsh National Boards for Nursing, Midwifery and Health Visiting in the 1980s (ENB courses 960 and 770, and their Welsh equivalents), academic developments in the early 1990s (diplomas in forensic care at Ashworth and Rampton Hospitals) and the publication of Working Paper 10 by the Department of Health in 1991 caused major changes in thinking about the workforce and its preparation for fitness to practise. The paradigm shifts associated with the NHS internal market and primary care-orientated services, the Reed Review of the early

1990s and the emergence of new epidemiological approaches to whole systems have led to a recognition of service deficits and have helped to unify the profession in a manner that has focused forensic nursing endeavours on the requirement to better influence policy and on the needs of service users.

This book is very much about policy and strategy developments in the 1990s – commencing with the Reed Review – and the implementation of policy and strategy changes in developing services and clinical practice by forensic mental health nurses.

At the time of publishing, the state of forensic mental health nursing is dynamic and exciting. It is noticeable that UK forensic nurses are contributing regularly to national and international nursing conferences and multidisciplinary seminars. The relative innocence and enthusiasm characteristic of any new entity are also present, and whilst the methodological rigour and academic 'tightness' associated with mature professions is as yet present only in patches, the willingness to question, experiment, learn and share is everywhere.

This text represents a point in time for forensic nurses in which there is a feeling that everything is newly open to scrutiny and constructive criticism – or is being rediscovered – and in which the traditional reliance upon custom and practice is being replaced by a spirit of exploration. Within this general revisionist environment, different services and units are at differing stages of development and change, and this will be apparent to the reader. It is not our intention to provide a set of stereotypical essays but instead to provide a vehicle for contributors to present, through their personal styles, the triumphs and frustrations of forensic nurses in their places of employment. The chapters, taken together, display many convergent characteristices: a very real awareness that everyone is not starting from the same point; the knowledge that 'truth' has many faces; academic rigour characterised by detailed evidence-based argument through to the pragmatic assertions of those 'feeling the way' (and making mistakes!) for others to follow; and an insight into excellence as yesterday's innovation. The chapters offer contradictions and different views of reality and paradigms. This is where forensic mental health nurses 'are at'.

Paul Tarbuck
Barry Topping-Morris
Philip Burnard

June 1999

Chapter 1
Reflections on the Reed Review – a nursing perspective

JOHN PARRY

The invitation to be a member of the Steering Group for the Reed Review (the Review of Health and Social Services for Mentally Disordered Offenders and Others Requiring Similar Services; Department of Health and Home Office, 1992) was both a learning experience and an opportunity to influence and debate the issues of care and service for mentally disordered offenders, not only with other disciplines, but also with other agencies at national levels. Since the publication of the Glancy Report (Department of Health, 1975) and Butler Report (Home Office and Department of Health and Social Security, 1975), many developments and changes have taken place within the NHS and other caring agencies. The Regional Secure Unit (RSU) programme has developed, albeit much more slowly than expected, together with the running down of large psychiatric hospitals and the reprovision of psychiatric services. Because of these developments, and in light of research for the Home Office by Gunn et al (1991), and of the Woolf Report (Home Office, 1991) into disturbances in the prison system, it was time to take stock of services nationally, and to provide recommendations for future developments.

In 1991, it was agreed that a joint Review be undertaken involving both the Department of Health and the Home Office. This joint arrangement was in itself a recognition of the importance of the Review and the increasing profile that mentally disordered people were beginning to receive. For so long, psychiatry had been seen as a 'Cinderella' service, and here was an opportunity to examine, on a national scale, the level and appropriateness of services to this group of the population.

It was particularly pleasing that the terms of reference for the Review included 'both health and social services for mentally disordered offenders and others who require similar services'. Those of us involved in forensic psychiatry and the provision of care within secure environments are aware that our provision is but one part of the continuum of care and range of services required by mentally disordered offenders (MDOs). Indeed, many regional NHS forensic services already provide community care in liaison with other agencies as the provision of adequate follow-up after discharge and early prevention of relapse are as important as inpatient care and treatment.

Membership of the Steering Group, whose role was to guide the Department of Health and the Home Office in the Review, reflected the variety of disciplines and agencies involved in the care and supervision of MDOs. Members came from the diverse agencies and professions associated with the care of MDOs, including representatives from the NHS – psychiatrists, nurses, service commissioners, finance officers and health authority members; Home Office and criminal justice system representatives – from the police, probation and prisons; and social service agency representatives – social workers. The involvement of health service commissioners and finance people indicated the anticipated resource implications arising from the Review.

Review strategy

At the first meeting of the Review in January 1992, the group realised how wide ranging the Review would be. A review of health service provision alone would have provided sufficient work for the group, but to include both social service provision and the implications of prison health care was a considerable challenge. The patient group included not only MDOs (already clearly associated with forensic psychiatry), but also offenders who had psychiatric problems and required health and social services input. This additionally included those patients who would be categorised as potential offenders, particularly those who posed a considerable risk to others in the community and in hospital.

Following considerable debate, three main areas of review were articulated:

- inpatient hospital care and treatment;
- community care and follow-up (by not only the health services, but also all the other agencies involved);
- psychiatric care and assessment within the prison system.

Three advisory groups were set up, formed from members of the Steering Group, each chaired by an officer from the Department of Health or the Home Office. Members of the Steering Group gave their preferences to serve on the advisory groups according to their area of work and expertise. Each advisory group met separately and reported back to the full Steering Group. Members of the Department and Home Office secretariat were allocated to each group and provided draft written reports.

Hospital Advisory Group

The Hospital Advisory Group reviewed the provision of high and medium security available at the time and took account of published and unpublished reports from the Department of Health (1990) and Special Hospitals Service Authority (1991), and a variety of published materials including those by Bluglass (1978), Faulk (1985), Gostin (1985) and Snowden (1990). There were indications that some patients in high security could be adequately managed in conditions of lesser security. The number of medium secure places (602 in January 1992) was well short of the initial Glancy target of 1000 nationally. The provision of low secure beds at local level fell from 1163 in 1956 to 639 in 1991 according to regional health authority returns. Whilst the late 1970s and early 80s had seen an increase in medium secure provision within the RSU programme, this coincided with the gradual closure of the large psychiatric hospitals and the redevelopment of psychiatric services in the community and local district general hospitals. There was anecdotal evidence of a need for longer-term medium security and more local secure provision.

Basson and Woodhouse (1985) and O'Grady (1990) described local secure provision in inner city areas and the importance of locked wards in meeting local needs. Reasons for admission included absconding, violence towards others and suicidal intent. In terms of general policy, patients referred to RSUs are thought to be a potential risk to others. However, many local services do not have locked facilities for all types of patient so some may be admitted to medium security provision in lieu of local secure facilities. There was clearly a need for a more factual picture of psychiatric provision at local level, and it was proposed that members of the Review would visit regions around the country to ascertain both provision and demand. This led to a recommendation, later in the Review, for local needs assessment on a regional basis rather than epidemiologically based norms for bed provision and services.

It was evident that the standards of skill mix and nurse-to-patient ratios set by the earlier RSUs had a profound effect on bed availability as services developed. Nursing involvement in the multidisciplinary assessment of patients referred to medium secure provision gave the profession greater involvement in and influence over admissions and bed occupancy, providing safe practice and good-quality care. Resources did not allow for this to be duplicated at local level.

The provision of high security was already under scrutiny at the time of the Review under the Chairmanship of Sir Louis Blom-Cooper, whose report was published in 1992. Because of the special nature of high secure care (including direct political interests), it was decided to recommend a further Working Group to report on the national provision and make recommendations for the future.

The recommendations of the Hospital Advisory Group reflected the gaps in service provision and ways in which these could be rectified. Local multiagency needs assessment, the availability of local locked wards and an increase in longer-term medium secure provision were the main themes. Other overlapping issues such as finance and resources, education and training were proposed for further debate later in the Review. The deliberations of the three advisory groups often overlapped in content, common themes arising within each group. A number of guiding principles emerged that applied to all MDOs throughout this spectrum of care. These were that patients should be cared for:

- with regard to the quality of care and proper attention to the needs of the individual;
- as far as possible in the community rather than in institutional settings;
- under conditions of no greater security than is justified by the degree of danger they present to themselves or others;
- in such a way as to maximise rehabilitation and their chances of sustaining an independent life;
- as near as possible to their own homes or families if they have them.

Community Advisory Group

The Community Advisory Group examined the complex and diverse services for mentally disordered offenders in the community (Figure 1.1). The terms of reference of the Review included offenders and potential offenders, many of whom were cared for in general psychiatry, community psychiatry and local social services. These broadly included:

- those diverted before entry into the criminal justice system;
- those discharged from hospital or released from prison;
- non-offenders who are vulnerable in the community, who may need assistance to prevent their offending, or may require access to a similar range of services.

The Advisory Group sought examples of good practice and models of service, such as duty psychiatrist schemes, assessment panel schemes, interagency working, community psychiatric nurse (CPN) diversion schemes, the Public Interest Case Assessment Project (PICA) and other pilot projects and research programmes. It was clear that the essential ingredient for good practice involved interagency collaboration, particularly at local level. The involvement of general psychiatry with MDOs is essential, and the most effective diversion schemes involve local mental health services, social services, local courts, the police and other agencies. The CPN – or community mental health nurse, to use the recently recommended title – has an increasing role to play as key worker ensuring continuity of care in the community and in developing models of practice. In 1990, the Home Office, in its Circular No. 66/90, gave details and recommendations to judges, courts, the police, the probation service and prison medical officers regarding their powers in dealing with MDOs and emphasised the increasing profile of and government concern over this group of patients.

Prison Advisory Group

The Prison Advisory Group had the benefit of recent reports into aspects of the prison medical services (Home Office, 1990a) and suicide and self-harm (Home Office, 1990b) as well as unpublished research by Gunn et al (1991) and Dell et al (1991). The Group endorsed, within their recommendations, the proposals for the prison service to contract in specialist mental health services. A number of standards were recommended for the assessment and care of prisoners with mental health needs. There is evidence, since the Review, that the recruitment of qualified mental health nurses into the prison service is increasing, and this presents a new challenge to the profession of nursing.

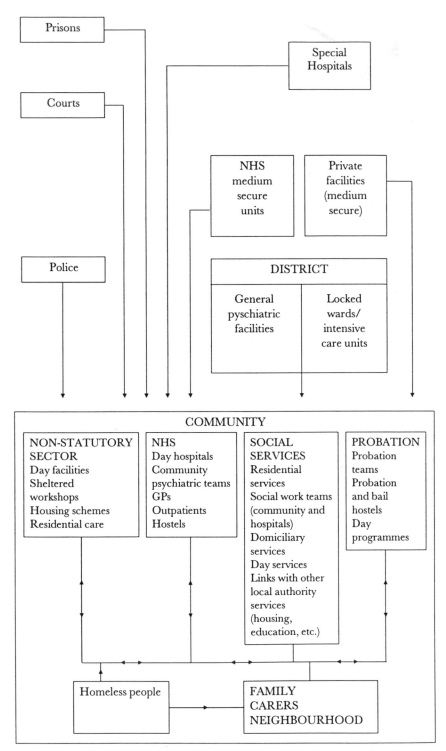

Figure 1.1. Mentally disordered offenders: sources of discharge or release into the community

Interim Report and further work

Following the reports of the Advisory Groups to the full Steering Committee, it was decided to publish an interim report on the progress of the Review. This outlined the work of the Advisory Groups, and their recommendations, giving an indication of further work to be done. There was considerable expectancy from staff working within forensic services of radical solutions and recommendations for change. At the time, some commentators said that many of the recommendations were 'statements of the obvious' and expressed some disappointment in the work of the Review. However, it was important to recognise in the Interim Report that models of good practice already existed and that gaps in service provision had been identified.

Interestingly, the work of the Review was being closely monitored by government ministers as the Review progressed. The Chairman and departmental officers were able to inform the Steering Group of ministerial interest on a continuing basis, and the style and format of reports drafted by the secretariat was very impressive. This did not restrict the views of the Steering Group members but gave a wider political dimension to its deliberations. Ministers emphasised that action would not be delayed unnecessarily while the Review was in progress and issued press releases to sustain the Review's momentum.

The Interim Report outlined a second wave of major issues arising from previous work. Groups were formed to consider finance, staffing, training and research. Other discrete areas of work included performance measurement and quality control and services for people with special needs.

Finance Advisory Group

Finance and resource issues pervaded many of the discussions about future service development. The Finance Advisory Group made recommendations regarding the planning of future services and the importance of identifying costs through needs assessment and the contracting process between purchasers and providers. Many of the proposals involved the better use of existing resources and ways of reducing costs by early intervention and improved collaboration between the agencies involved in delivering care. However, it was recognised that hospital services (particularly an increase in secure provision) would require additional funding, and allocations of capital monies were made available during the course of the Review. An important aspect of purchasing, given the financial disincentives for health authorities to address the needs of patients in the Special Hospital system, was the recommendation that 'Districts should, as a medium term aim, become responsible for obtaining high security provision for their residents, but this should be within a framework that ensures continued availability of an adequate number of high security places nationally' (Recommendation 5.39, Report of the Finance Advisory Group). Information on Special Hospital costs attributable to their residents was already becoming available to the health authorities, but it was recognised that there needed to be a financial incentive to transfer patients from high secure care when clinically appropriate.

Workforce, education and training

Service provision for MDOs involves many staff groups, including health care professionals, social and probation services, prison health care staff, therapists and others. The Staffing and Training Groups identified the staffing requirements necessary to meet the increased number of secure beds. Other staffing needs, it recommended, should reflect the level and pattern of local services determined by needs assessment and quality requirements. As with the other staff groups, the onus was placed upon employers to consider the implications of nurse staffing and training, in light of the recommendations, and, in conjunction with nurse training centres, jointly to plan training to meet development requirements. Training and placements for CPNs in forensic psychiatry were recommended, and proposals were made for the English National Board for Nursing, Midwifery and Health Visiting (ENB) to consider the future need for Project 2000 training in forensic nursing. The targeting of post-basic courses in forensic nursing on a wider group of nursing staff (other than those working in high and medium secure settings) was recognised as a useful mechanism to increase the skills base and awareness of the workforce.

Research implications

The importance of research in informing and improving future practice received considerable emphasis in the recommendations. Recommended research priorities are outlined in the Report (Table 1.1), and this area presents a major challenge for nursing staff working within forensic psychiatry. Much expertise and information is already available, and this could be shared to much greater effect by research publications and professional forums. The formation of the national forensic nursing database (see Chapter 16) is exactly what the Review was advocating. The importance of academic development was addressed in the Review, with recommendations for the Department of Health and Home Office to consider an increase in the number of academic posts to cover forensic psychiatry, child and adolescent psychiatry, and learning disabilities. Regional forensic advisers were proposed to help to develop a national strategy for academic development, and Recommendation 11.229 stated that 'the academic base for forensic nursing should be expanded within a structured multi-disciplinary framework'.

Advisory Group on Special Needs

It was recognised that there were a number of patient groups who, within existing services, did not have sufficient provision or priority. The Advisory Group on Special Needs made recommendations regarding these groups, which include persons with learning disabilities, autism and brain injury, children and adolescents, substance misusers, women, those from small ethnic groups, sex offenders with mental health needs and other groups that, although small in number, are entitled to improved provision.

Final Summary Report

The work of the Review was completed in mid-1992, having taken 18 months. Reports from the various Advisory Groups were published, along with the Interim Report in 1991 and the Final Report in 1992. This amounted to 11 separate reports in all, addressing the issues outlined in this chapter. Because of the volume of work and documentation, the Final Report summarised the work of the Review and set out all the 276 recommendations made throughout the Review. However, there were two remaining issues that required further in-depth examination, namely high-security provision and psychopathic disorder. Although these issues were addressed during the Review, it was clear that further time was needed to examine the possible major implications of changes and developments in these areas of service. Two further working parties were set up under the Chairmanship of Dr John Reed to report back in a further 6 months.

Conclusions

Over the past 15 or more years, the most noticeable development in services for MDOs has been, along with the growth in services, the multidisciplinary teamworking approach. This was reflected in the

Table 1.1. Possible components of a strategic plan for research on mentally disordered offenders

Topic	Social policy	Basic research in medicine, etc.	Service delivery	Legal and penal practice
Mentally disordered offenders	Relationships between prevalence of offending by mentally disordered and social deprivation	Epidemiological surveys by NHS Region Longitudinal studies of MDOs Development of drug treatments	Provision of services by general psychiatrists Quality of aftercare in community	Use of hospital/guardianship/probation orders or prison sentences
Personality disorders	Environmental factors that influence personality disorder	*Literature review *Treatability issues *Diagnostic issues	*Evaluation of treatment	Use of hospital/prison disposals
Sexual offenders		*Distinction between sexual disorders and sexual offending Epidemiological survey in UK	*Roles of penal health and social services	Effect of changes in law
Violent offenders	Effect on victims	Relation to mental disorder Treatment programmes in prison and community	Evaluation of treatment programmes	
Police		Profiling offenders	*Services required to assist police to identify MDOs	*Use of Section 136
Community services		Effect of the reprovision of local services on mental health	*Effect of social supervision of restricted patients	
Prisoners		*Prevalence of mental disorder in the remand prison population	Arrangements for mental health services for prisoners	Measures to prevent suicide or self-harm

Table 1.1. (contd)

Topic	Social policy	Basic research in medicine, etc.	Service delivery	Legal and penal practice
Adolescents	Effect of disturbed childhood on later incidence of mental disorder/offending	Indicators of future offending (especially sexual offending)	Evaluation of current interventions (especially sexual offending)	Pathways into custody of juveniles (effects of new child and criminal justice legislation)
Diversion	Attitudes of prison officers to MDOs; Public attitude to not prosecuting mentally disordered offenders		*Resources required for effective diversion schemes	MHA sections – suitability of, for diverting MDOs from criminal system; Power of judges/magistrates
Hospital services	*Outcome indicators for hospital care		*Assessment of needs for different types of hospital provision	
Women		Prevalence of mental disorder	Availability/use of services	Differential use of hospital orders
Ethnic minorities		*Evaluation of treatment approaches and responses	*Availability/use of services; *Equitable treatment of ethnic minorities	

MDOs = mentally disordered offenders; MHA = Mental Health Act.
*Recommended priority (RS 6.8).

constitution of the Review Steering Group. The willingness of differing agencies to work together was a sign of the experience and maturity attained to date and boded well for increased co-operation in the future. Nursing, as a profession, was recognised as a major contributor to the process of the Review and an influence in the planning and development of future services. The opportunities for nursing are clear: members of the profession must ensure that they are involved at all levels of decision-making about service provision for MDOs. The sense of teamwork and collaboration was a major theme of the Reed Review and calls for considerable flexibility in approach when working together to provide improved services in the future. It is confidently expected that the nursing profession and other professionals and agencies will rise to the challenge.

References

Basson JV, Woodhouse M (1985) Assessment of a secure/intensive care/forensic ward. Acta Psychiatrica Scandinavica 64: 132–41.

Blom-Cooper L (1992) Report of the Committee of Inquiry into Complaints about Ashworth Hospital, Volume 2. London: HMSO.

Bluglass R (1978) Regional secure units and interim security for psychiatric patients. British Medical Journal 1: 489–483.

Dell S, Grounds A, James K, Robertson G (1991) Mentally Disordered Remand Prisoners: Report to the Home Office. London: Home Office.

Department of Health (1975) Report on Security in NHS Hospitals (The Glancy Report). London: HMSO.

Department of Health (1990) Regional Returns on RSU Beds. Internal report. London: Department of Health.

Department of Health and Home Office (1992) Review of Health and Social Services for Mentally Disordered Offenders and Others Requiring Similar Services (The Reed Review). Cmnd 2088. London: HMSO.

Faulk M (1985) Basic Forensic Psychiatry. London: Blackwell Scientific Publications.

Gostin L (1985) Secure Provision: A Review of Special Services for the Mentally Ill and Mentally Handicapped in England and Wales 1985. London: Tavistock Publications.

Gunn J, Maden A, Swinton M (1991) The Number of Psychiatric Cases Among Sentenced Prisoners – Report to the Home Office. London: Home Office.

Home Office (1990a) Report on an Efficiency Scrutiny of the Prison Medical Service. London: Home Office.

Home Office (1990b) Report on a Review by Her Majesty's Chief Inspector of Prisons – Suicide and Self Harm in the Prison Service Establishments in England and Wales. Cmnd 1383. London: HMSO.

Home Office (1991) Report on Prison Disturbances – April 1990 (The Woolf Report). Cmnd 1456. London: HMSO.

Home Office and Department of Health and Social Security (1975) Report of the Committee on Mentally Abnormal Offenders (The Butler Report). Cmnd 6244. London: HMSO.

O'Grady J (1990) The complementary roles of regional and local secure provision for psychiatric patients. Health Trends 22(1).

Snowden P (1990) Regional secure units and forensic services in England and Wales. In Bluglass R, Bowden P (Eds) Practice of Forensic Psychiatry. London: Churchill Livingstone.

Special Hospitals Service Authority (1991) Within Maximum Security Hospitals: A Survey of Need. Unpublished report. London: SHSA.

Chapter 2
The forensic multidisciplinary care team

STEPHEN BURROW

The multidisciplinary ethos is now established at a time when there has been a substantial development of a broad range of professional health care groups. The most basic definition of a multidisciplinary clinical team was that of:

> a group of colleagues acknowledging a common involvement in the care and treatment of a particular patient. (Royal Commission, 1979)

Teamwork is viewed as an integral part of health care delivery because the client group manifests such a range of health and social needs. Obviously, no one individual, of whatever discipline, can implement such a varied programme of care for individual patients. Instead, the discrete skills of individual experts must be co-ordinated to serve the patient's best interests (Evers, 1981) to produce a 'negotiated order' amongst integrated health care disciplines (Evers, 1977) and, by effecting collaborative working, to constitute good practice. Certainly, the nurses' Code of Professional Conduct (UKCC, 1993), for example, statutorily prescribes that they should recognise, and co-operate with, other health care agencies and enhance the reputation of other 'professions', implying the interrelationship and interdependence of the various professional groups. At the same time, each of the professional groups – as quite separate bodies – has a duty of care to its clients and must act within the limits of its own occupational boundaries. In the case of nursing, each individual is held personally accountable for his or her professional practice by the Code of Professional Conduct. So, far from metamorphosing into one rational, harmonious partnership, the diverse membership of the multidisciplinary team has the potential for considerable conflict.

Team leadership and responsibility

Interdisciplinary conflict in the team setting is documented in terms of: role, leadership and team objectives (Milne, 1993); clinical responsibility and independence, and the protection of territorial boundaries (Appleyard and Maden, 1979; Fairhurst, 1977); the conflict of clinical goals and priorities (Strauss et al, 1963); the organisational difficulties and complexity of managing teams (Guy, 1986); and, with specific reference to nurses and doctors, disputes over professional care, management responsibilities and patients' rights (Diamond, 1987). Leadership of the team is seen to lie with medical staff in some quarters (Appleyard and Maden, 1979; British Geriatrics Society and Royal College of Nursing, 1975; Department of Health and Social Security, 1975; Hodkinson, 1975). Alternative views suggest that there should be corporate responsibility for the clinical area (Morgan, 1993; South East Thames Regional Health Authority, 1976); that any one professional may take 'prime responsibility' for a client (Milne, 1993); and that the sharing of leadership functions utilises team members' abilities rather than demanding compliance (Margerison and McCann, 1986; Milne, 1993).

Historical perspective

Historically, psychiatric institutions were dominated by the medical superintendent, who had authority over every hospital professional group, including social work, nursing and administration. The strength of his domination not only ranged over hospital affairs, but also included social matters such as the need for nursing staff to seek his permission before marrying. The fact that individuals from within hospital or treatment teams contributed their technical skills did not undermine the almost regal authority of the superintendent. The psychiatric sector, for example, could call upon the services of the psychologist, psychiatric social worker, occupational therapist, nurse, chaplain and industrial officer. It was not expected that these representatives would regularly collaborate as focused teams other than in individual cases, but that they would operate more as a hospital network of potential services. Gradually, a growing commitment emerged towards developing multiprofessional collaboration, which provided an ongoing potential for 'specialist therapeutic teams', especially primary care teams in the community (Department of Health and Social Security, 1975). An increasing influx of psychologists and social workers was viewed as helping to constitute the multidisciplinary approach to care, reduce the restrictive atmosphere of the hospital and replace the 'tightly controlled medical culture' (Nolan, 1993).

Considerable impetus was given to the establishment of multiprofessional teams in psychiatric care by the Committee of Enquiry into St Augustine's Hospital. Having investigated allegations about the treatment and care of patients, it recommended the instigation of multidisciplinary teams at hospital, clinical area and ward levels on the basis that:

> the most effective organisations are likely to be those where there is parity of esteem between the professions. (South East Thames Regional Health Authority, 1976)

The purposes of multidisciplinary teams

Many of the foregoing issues have manifested themselves in the forensic psychiatric field. Yet it was for precisely the type of advantage accruing from 'focusing the activities and expertise of the various professions' that the Butler Committee recommended the establishment of a national network of medium secure units to manage a certain proportion of the mentally disordered group of clients (Home Office and Department of Health and Social Security, 1975). The concentration of forensic psychiatric services at these centres would provide comprehensive assessments – psychiatric, psychological, social and nursing – of any mental abnormality of clients who had been referred by the courts. These clients would also benefit from the range of treatments provided by such a team, who would provide a concerted reference point for the probation and aftercare service when in need of advice.

This fresh start did not have the pervasive effect on more established forensic institutions that it might have had. The traditional network – termed Special Hospitals – have a statutory role to manage patients who have a propensity for violence, in conditions of special security. In 1988, one such establishment – Broadmoor Hospital – following an inspection of its services, was heavily criticised for the underdevelopment of multidisciplinary collaboration and teamwork commitment. The report proposed that 'therapeutic enthusiasm' was generated by teamworking and care-planning even though 'some responsibilities fall naturally to individual professionals', 'sometimes with a single professional taking the lead' (NHS Advisory Service and DHSS Social Services Inspectorate, 1988). Yet, more recently, the Ashworth Inquiry, investigating complaints into that hospital, noted that when non-nursing staff visited the wards, they were so marginalised that they were entered into the ward documentation along with any other 'visitors'. The authors commented that 'suspicion, hostility and ownership appear to be insurmountable obstacles' to multidisciplinary working (Department of Health and Speical Hospitals Service Authority, 1992).

One of the most recent multidisciplinary initiatives to be forwarded derived from the deliberations of the Reed Review, which recommended a 'multi-professional core team' to assess MDOs 'at the point of entry' into the forensic health service and ensured their referral to the appropriate setting (Department of Health and Home Office, 1991). The role of multidisciplinary collaboration in the management of forensic patients' needs is now irreversibly established. The process has progressed to the point of formulating collaborative care-planning, which, it is hoped, will reach the level of sophistication to identify 'critical pathways', and individual disciplines and their attendant interventions, during the anticipated course of treatment.

But in what ways do the services provided by the forensic team generate distinctive problems additional to those already outlined? A forensic focus in health care relates to a therapeutic targeting of any aspect of a patient's behaviour that links his or her psychiatric symptomatology and offending behaviour (Burrow, 1993a). This offending behaviour can take the form of any illegal activity but, at its most extreme, may relate to:

> unprovoked or random physical or sexual assaults on members of the public; psychotic symptoms which involve specific people, with or without threats, which could lead to the commission of violent acts; arson; the use of poison or drugs to cause harm to others; the use of firearms, knives, explosive devices, missile and other weapons; sadistic behaviour; hostage-taking; and persistent scheming or determined absconding in the context of harmful or potentially harmful behaviour. (Gunn and Taylor, 1993)

Clearly, patients exhibiting such behaviours in the context of mental disorder are not politely invited voluntarily to participate in treatment, often within secure institutions!

Members of the team as expert witnesses

Allocation to treatment facilities will, largely, but not exclusively, be by involuntary legal disposal following the court appearance of defendants apprehended for their offences. This throws up a number of related impediments for forensic disciplines. First, some of the disciplines – predominantly psychiatrists, social workers and psychologists – are used by the courts to provide expert witness reports about defendants. This can be seen to be wholly beneficial in the case of those whose illness is so incapacitating that they are unfit even to stand trial, or those whose disorder acquits them of responsibility for their actions. However, it has been argued that, in other respects, such involvement compromises the therapeutic basis of a health care role (Diamond, 1990, 1992; Stone, 1984). Far from operating solely as a client-advocate, such a role is indubitably that of a 'hired hand', performed, first and foremost, on behalf of the criminal justice system, which attempts to determine a defendant's criminal culpability. Put most succinctly:

> the task is not healing, but evaluation for the purpose of testimony in court to advance the general interests of justice. (Appelbaum, 1990)

Consequently, health care professionals, in their capacity as expert witnesses to the court, derive their information about a client on the basis of the confidential relationship existing between doctor and patient, only to exhibit it before criminal justice professionals within the court process. Such information may then be advertised via media to which the entire general public has inevitable access, especially if it documents homicide or other attention-grabbing events.

In another respect, the most potentially disconcerting aspect of a 'successful' diversion of the MDO to a psychiatric hospital is the potential for this becoming an indefinite life sentence. In contrasting this with the more or less definitive term of a criminal conviction, one becomes aware of the potential for the health witness to extend the custodial life of the 'patient'.

Expert witness contributions by health professionals also involve recommendations of 'treatability', which is an effort to determine which patients might respond favourably to given environments and modes of treatment. Treatability is, therefore, a concept of clinical potential. On the other hand, many professionals surmise that the courts prioritise public safety rather than individual patients' mental state. It could be argued, therefore, that the thrust of the treatability evaluation is predicting future dangerousness, which is highly problematic because of the severity of the mental disorder, the relatedness of the offending behaviour to the illness, and the responsiveness of patients to treatment. The conclusion is that, subject to such complex variables, treatment is unlikely to have a major effect on thwarting patient recidivism. Nevertheless, in the commissioner–

provider contractual climate, there will be an increasing pressure on forensic teams to anticipate treatment outcomes for individual clients.

Risk assessment by the team

A main component of the discussions between service commissioner and provider will inevitably concern the risk assessment and management plan for the client that has been constructed by the multidisciplinary team. Risk assessment entails generating an understanding of the potential reoffending of the client and the nature of the client's propensities. The political profile of the offending activities, cause forensic disciplines to be orientated towards predicting and precluding dangerousness. All health agents acting for MDOs are compelled to regard the forensic history of clients at least as seriously as issues related to their psychiatric diagnoses. The assembled team have to negotiate their individual interventions and perceptions while, simultaneously, acknowledging the ongoing contribution of their colleagues, who may unearth some previously hidden client trait that may constitute a risk. Indeed, the very safety of the patient and staff community, as well as visitors and external public, may very well depend on a shared and consistent agreement about how to tackle the risks and issues relating to particular individuals.

It is unlikely that anything but a collaborative approach will reveal all of the details and circumstances that provoked and precipitated a client's mental deterioration and offending. Nor can a successful prospect of future client stability be remotely guaranteed without a pooling of interdisciplinary perceptions of risk. Forensic health care demands a professional rigour that focuses largely on what constitutes an acceptable treatment risk correlated with the possible adverse consequences of endangering the safety of the general public. Managing such contentious variables is bound to produce unexpected outcomes, sometimes emanating from erroneous judgements and leading to absconding, escape, hostage-taking, serious assault and even manslaughter, for example.

The multidisciplinary team and security

This necessitates that all staff, particularly those of the multidisciplinary care team, engage in a security role that affects them at interpersonal, environmental and technological levels. In turn, the higher the level of institutional security, the greater the potential dilution of a therapeutic climate by custodial policies. For team members functioning in high-security Special Hospitals, a spate of high-profile abscondings potentiated the routine application of security procedures. In addition to established strategies – the investigation of most patients' mail, the photographing of all patients, and environmental safety checks – any temporary absence of a patient from the hospital will demand absolute continuous observation at all times, the searching of the patients' clothes beforehand and the need to consider the application of handcuffs. Such policies clearly generate peculiar opportunities for team schisms as organisational imperatives challenge professional sensitivities on the one hand, and individual members debate these contingencies on the other. Consequently, patient care is not discussed in isolation from a wider remit including unit policies on admissions, discharges, ward routines and staff numbers needed for patient trips, for example. Although operational guidelines may erect a security shroud over a particular institution, this should not preclude individual teams from adapting these when appropriate.

The environment for team decision-making

To complicate matters further, affirmations of multidisciplinary collaboration are required to be negotiated amongst a web of other superstructural agencies. Highly respected health care and human rights groups such as MIND, the Community Health Council, the Consumers Advice Bureau, Women in Special Hospitals and hospital advisory committees, enter the general fray on behalf of clients. On the other hand, the Home Office might refuse months of interagency efforts to organise a client's trial rehabilitation programme on the grounds that this represents a disproportionate risk. Patient discharge decisions may be objected to by the Home Office Advisory Board, whose remit is to assess the criminal propensity of clients despite evidence of their improved mental state. Conversely, Mental Health Review Tribunals may decide not to heed the team's long-standing deliberations and reservations about an individual client's discharge.

Riley (1991) warns against the assumption that multiprofessional psychiatric agencies share a common philosophy and has contrasted the traditional model of practitioner domination with that of the emerging facilitative empowerment of consumers. If this situation prevails in the 'community' climate, how much more likely are there to be schisms in the forensic team who address the contentious issues surrounding the MDO? The trend toward the client-focused care of forensic patients is certainly not necessarily shared by either the public or all mental health practitioners. It generates unique contradictions and dilemmas, particularly for nursing staff (Burrow, 1991, 1993b; Department of Health, 1994). Whilst there will probably always be team dissension about the clinical management of individuals, it is equally highly likely that these overlie hugely divergent values with respect to the patient group and their repatriation, or otherwise, to society.

Research and the multidisciplinary perspective

Whilst there has been an increase in the literature, including research, on forensic health care by individual disciplines, there have been few truly multidisciplinary collaborations. Multidisciplinary research is very much on the political and professional agenda (Department of Health, 1994). One such paper described the concerted effort to establish a unit for individuals with 'psychopathic disorder' at Broadmoor Hospital (Brett, 1992). The venture outlined the group-orientated regime, limitations and treatment objectives of a team that necessitated the collaboration of psychiatrists, a psychologist, a speech therapist, a psychotherapist, a patient-educationalist and nurses. The speech therapist, for example, was able to focus on language skills and difficulties in order to improve communication and, in turn, the group participation of clients.

A research project between the Department of Health and the Special Hospitals Service Authority brought together an academic, two psychiatrists, a psychologist and a nurse to investigate the treatment and security needs of patients in Special Hospitals (Burrow, 1993c; Maden et al, 1993). Without each other, none of the individual professions would have elicited the information that they did collectively. They elaborated on: client profiles; the unnecessarily high levels of security for between 35% and 50% of the client group; the nature of client deficits in addition to mental disorder and offending behaviour; the co-terminous as well as conflicting demands of both treatment and security features of care; and the strategic recommendation for a new tier of long-term, medium secure units for some MDOs and similarly placed people.

Shared vision and understanding

The advance of multidisciplinary health care necessarily incorporates an expansion of therapeutic modes and their required skills, an overlapping of roles, conflicts concerning autonomy and independence, and tensions over team leadership within these groups. Articulating such diversity is constructively appraised by Griffin (1989), who recognised the advantages of a multidisciplinary collaboration that prescribes 'full clinical responsibility' for the consultant or general practitioner, 'independent professional responsibility' for each team member, and 'shared responsibility' for decisions taken by all team members together' (Department of Health and Social Security, 1977).

Additionally, as West (1989) suggests, it is necessary, in relation to any teamwork: to share a vision of what is to be achieved; to provide for decision-making opportunities for all members; to focus on an improving, quality service; and to gain managerial support for resources and time for collaboration. It should be a priority to tackle structural impediments in order to counteract interdisciplinary alienation such as prevailed at Ashworth Hospital, where the geographically dispersed wards effectively created a constellation of separate, satellite facilities (Rae, 1993), so that even other team personnel were identified as 'visitors' on ward documentation.

Conclusions

The development away from a medical domination towards a more democratic model of interdisciplinary involvement in clinical decision-making has aimed at achieving a higher standard of patient care irrespective of the health field. However, teams managing MDOs cannot simply focus exclusively on an improved clinical care package. The forensic team has unique concerns that demand even greater efforts at effective collaboration. It also has an implicit social control remit that predominantly custodialises MDOs, targets offence behaviour related to psychiatric morbidity, and unavoidably adopts security practices within and outside secure institutions for the purpose of maintaining a climate of universal safety. Furthermore, to a greater degree than in most health fields, concerted team planning may be compromised or refashioned by non-clinical agencies. The operational imperative for such groups is not merely the need for even greater collaborative integrity in producing a consensus on individual patient planning. Because of the wide-ranging repercussions that can be generated by the care of forensic clients, it is indispensable for the forensic team to pool ongoing assessment, therapeutic intervention, holistic client management, expert advice, training and education. The 'Achilles heel' for the forensic team is that, however conscientiously they refine, co-ordinate and celebrate their professional practice, their performance will always be pressurised by non-clinical constraints and be judged by the incidence of client recidivism. It is then the role of organisational managers to play their part in the team by supporting clinical decision-making in addition to instituting mechanisms that address any shortfalls in the process.

On his or her part, the insightful client is all too aware that every detail of behaviour is continuously scrutinised, not only on the client's behalf, but also on that of fellow patients, staff, relatives and the wider community. Even behaviour illustrating dissension from treatment may be interpreted in an unfavourable and potentially dangerousness light. In such circumstances, there is every incentive for the forensic client to attempt to conceal any deviant symptom from his or her treatment team in the knowledge that it may well delay a return to normal life. The team's objective in such circumstances is to engage patients' trust by encouraging participation in, and evaluation of, their personal care as well as in decision-making about issues that directly affect them as service users. Notwithstanding this, there can be no denial that current team intentions are tempered by the harsh facts of history.

References

Applebaum PS (1990) The parable of the forensic psychiatrist: ethics and the problem of doing harm. International Journal of Law and Psychiatry 13: 249–59.

Appleyard J, Maden JG (1979) Multidisciplinary teams. British Medical Journal 2(6200): 1305–7.

Brett T (1992) Treatment in Secure Hospitals. Criminal Behaviour and Mental Health, 2(2): 152–58.

British Geriatrics Society and Royal College of Nursing (1975) Improving Geriatric Care in Hospital. London: RCN.

Burrow S (1991) The special hospital nurse and the dilemma of therapeutic custody. Journal of Advances in Health and Nursing Care 1(3): 21–38.

Burrow S (1993a) An outline of the forensic nursing role. British Journal of Nursing 2(18): 899–904.

Burrow S (1993b) The role conflict of the forensic nurse. Senior Nurse 13(5): 20–5.

Burrow S (1993c) The treatment and security needs of special hospital patients – a nursing perspective. Journal of Advanced Nursing 18: 1267–78.

Department of Health (1994) Working in Partnership. London: HMSO.

Department of Health and Home Office (1991) Review of Health and Social Services for Mentally Disordered Offenders and Others Requiring Similar Services (The Reed Review). Cmnd 2088. London: HMSO.

Department of Health and Social Security (1975) Better Services for the Mentally Ill. London: HMSO.

Department of Health and Social Security (1977) The Role of Psychologists in the Health Services: Report of the Sub-Committee (Chairman: Professor WH Trethowan). London: HMSO.

Department of Health and Special Hospitals Service Authority (1992) Report of the Committee of Inquiry into Complaints about Ashworth Hospital, Vols I and II. Cmnd 2028. London: HMSO.

Diamond BL (1987) Your disobedient servant. Nursing Times 83(4): 28–31.

Diamond BL (1990) The psychiatrist expert witness: honest advocate or 'hired gun'? In Rosner R, Weistock R (Eds) Ethical Practice in Psychiatry and the Law. New York: Plenum Press.

Diamond BL (1992) The forensic psychiatrist: consultant vs. activist in legal doctrine. Bulletin of the American Academy of Psychiatry and the Law 20: 119–32.

Evers HK (1977) The patient care team in the hospital ward: the place of the nursing student. Journal of Advanced Nursing 2: 589–96.

Evers HK (1981) Multidisciplinary teams in geriatric wards: myth or reality? Journal of Advanced Nursing 6: 205–14.

Fairhurst E (1977) Teamwork as Panacea: Some Underlying Assumptions. Unpublished Paper. Annual Conference of the Medical Sociology Group of the British Sociological Association, University of Warwick.

Griffin NV (1989) Multi-professional care in forensic psychiatry. Psychiatric Bulletin 13: 613–15.

Gunn J, Taylor P (1993) Forensic Psychiatry: Clinical, Legal and Ethical Issues. Oxford: Butterworth-Heinemann.

Guy ME (1986) Interdisciplinary conflict and organisational complexity. Hospital and Health Services Administration 31(1): 111–21.

Hodkinson HM (1975) An Outline of Geriatrics. London: Academic Press.

Home Office and Department of Health and Social Security (1975) Report of the Committee on Mentally Abnormal Offenders. Cmnd 6224. London: HMSO.

Maden A, Curle C, Meux C, Burrow S, Gunn J (1993) Treatment and Security Needs of Special Hospitals Patients. London: Whurr Publishers.

Margerison C, McCann D (1986) High performance management teams. Health Care Management 1(1): 26–31.

Milne D (1993) Psychology and Mental Health Nursing. London: Macmillan.

Morgan S (1993) Community Mental Health. London: Chapman & Hall.

NHS Advisory Service and DHSS Social Services Inspectorate (1988) Report on Services Provided by Broadmoor Hospital. London: Health Advisory Service.

Nolan P (1993) A History of Mental Health Nursing. London: Chapman & Hall.

Rae M (1993) Freedom to Care. Merseyside: Ashworth Hospital Graphics Department.

Riley M (1991) A collective responsibility. Nursing Standard 5(33): 18–20.

Royal Commission (1979) Royal Commission on the National Health Service. London: HMSO.

South East Thames Regional Health Authority (1976) Report of Committee of Enquiry into St. Augustine's Hospital, Chartham. London: HMSO.

Stone AA (1984) The ethical boundaries of forensic psychiatry: a view from the ivory tower. Bulletin of the American Academy of Psychiatry and the Law 12: 209–19.

Strauss A, Schatzman L, Ehrlich D, Bucher R, Sabshin M (1963) The Hospital and its Negotiated Order. In Freidson B (Ed.) The Hospital in Modern Society. London: Macmillan.

UKCC (United Kingdom Central Council for Nursing, Midwifery and Health Visiting) (1993) Code of Professional Conduct, 3rd Edn. London: UKCC.

West M (1989) Visions and team innovations. Reproduced in Milne D (1993) Psychology and Mental Health Nursing. London: Macmillan.

Chapter 3
The treatment, care and management of the psychopathic disorder patient: the nursing contribution

DAVID SALLAH

The term 'psychopathic disorder' has retained its presence in British psychiatry, obviously with a meaning and usefulness for clinicians, practitioners and the general public. The odd thing, however, is that it refers to a purely legal category associated with socially orientated controls rather than a medical diagnosis with treatment implications. The diagnosis of the condition often relates to the degree and extent of the behaviour that is seen as antisocial. Previous reviews of psychopathic disorder include those of the Percy Commission (Royal Commission, 1957), the Butler Committee (Home Office and Department of Health and Social Security, 1975) and the Department of Health and Social Security (1986), none of which has been very successful in identifying the best approach to the care, treatment and management of the sufferer. The Reed Review (Department of Health and Home Office, 1994) addressed the issue in its Working Group on the subject, with a view to identifying what methods of management and treatment are likely to be most effective. Significantly, and unlike the situation with psychopathic disorder, 'personality disorder' is defined in clinical terms and therefore has a host of traits with treatment options (American Psychiatric Association, 1980).

This chapter discusses some of the relevant issues, drawing on the deliberations of the Reed Review, and identifies the nursing contribution to the management of patients with psychopathic disorder. It also appeals for the redress of the apparent deficit in knowledge base throughout the professions, particularly nursing.

Definition of psychopathic disorder

The term 'psychopathic' literally means 'psychically damaged' and was introduced in the nineteenth century in Germany to cover all forms of psychopathology. In England and Wales, the Mental Health Act 1983 indicates psychopathic disorder to be:

> a persistent disorder or disability of mind (whether or not including significant impairment of intelligence) which results in abnormally aggressive or seriously irresponsible conduct on the part of the person concerned.

The difficulty with this definition is that it embraces a wide range of clinical conditions and therefore does not clarify which behaviour is best treated or managed and in which environment. The lack of any clinical definition of the term only reinforces the view among many professional staff that the legal definition only exists as a means of detaining people in secure hospitals and units.

What is almost universally agreed upon by clinicians and other practitioners alike is the fact that the diagnosis of psychopathic disorder is unreliable: there is disagreement on its definition, and its very usage has pejorative connotations for the general public. Furthermore, and quite regrettably, most clinicians use the term to describe a situation in which it is generally felt that the patient is incurable or untreatable (Gunn and Robertson, 1976). Another source of confusion is the growing use of the term 'personality disorder'. Although this is defined in clinical terms and has specific options for care and management, it is often substituted for the term 'psychopathic disorder', complicating approaches and attitudes to treatment, care and management. Because of this, there have been calls, not least from nurses, for the simplification and clarification of the terminology.

In a recent survey of nurses' views conducted to inform the Reed Review (Sallah, 1994), 59% of the respondents thought that the term 'psychopathic disorder' should be removed from the Mental Health Act 1983. This is not dissimilar to the views expressed by consultant forensic psychiatrists (Cope, 1993) also commissioned to inform the Review.

Diagnosing psychopathic disorder

Dolan and Coid (1993) argued that:

> little progress can be made in assessing the treatability of psychopaths or devising appropriate treatment programmes unless it is clear from the outset exactly what it is that is being treated.

Attempts have been made to classify the characteristics of the behaviour displayed by the psychopath (see, for example, Blackburn, 1986; Checkley, 1976; Hare, 1991). What is clear, however, is that psychopathic disorder is not a homogenous condition but requires a variety of approaches and treatment modalities, drawing on the skills and experiences of all the professionals who provide care for the sufferer.

Elsewhere in Europe, the Netherlands provides a model for the care of the MDO, particularly the psychopath. The model is organised through a system of hospital provisions – *Terbeschikkingstelling* (TBS). This loosely translates as placing a person in a secure hospital at the pleasure of the state and with restrictions on discharge, similar to the way in which Sections 37 and 41 of the Mental Health Act 1983 are applied. There is a variety of hospitals, or *Kinieken*, that are privately or publicly owned and are operated on a provision of care based on the specialist nature of that particular hospital. Patients are therefore placed in environments specialising in meeting their specific needs, rather than trying to fit them into an existing hospital (which may not be able to meet their needs effectively). The care in the private clinics is funded by the Justice Ministry and/or Health Ministry, or through private insurance. The telling question is whether or not the system allows for improved diagnostic advances and the subsequent treatment of the condition. The point, however, is that the Dutch are approaching the problem in a more co-ordinated manner.

The Dutch legal system – used for managing MDOs and especially those with psychopathic disorder – owes a great deal to the experiences of a number of civil servants, academics, lawyers and other professionals who were detained in prisons during World War II as political prisoners. They became acquainted with the plight of the other prisoners and the background to their offending behaviours. After the war, these political prisoners, some of whom were psychiatrists, decided that MDOs deserved to be located and cared for under conditions of security that concentrate on the health care needs of the individual. Thus, the post-war period was characterised by the search for an individual approach to criminal justice in general (Fick, 1947), a situation that resulted in a greater co-operation between the criminal justice system and the psychiatric services. For example, the chairs of forensic psychiatry fall within the Faculty of Law in Dutch universities, and legal professionals are on the staff of some of the TBS hospitals.

The system has two main sentencing approaches: *straffen* (punitive) and *maatregelen* (non-punitive). The punitive sentences contain an element of retribution (in most cases a prison sentence, thus depriving the individual of liberty) and precaution against future misdemeanour. The non-punitive sentences are for the protection of society from the offender, and where mental disorder is seen to be a contributory factor in respect of the crime, a psychiatrist's opinion is sought to help the judge to make a decision. A non-punitive judgement may include a TBS order, which may last for as long as the judge thinks that the person is still a danger to society, the individual being kept in a mental institution legally identified as suitable for the treatment and management of the problem presented by the individual. This may last longer than the defined sentence for the crime committed. The punitive and non-punitive options may benefit from inputs from the health care sector.

A TBS order may be made for any crime as long as there is evidence of mental disorder, and for all crimes that attract a maximum sentence of 4 years. This can be extended beyond the 4 years if the crime was of a violent nature and endangered other people, or for reasons of public safety. There is an appeal after the first year of the extension period. If there is the need to extend the order beyond 6 years in total, the judge must seek expert advice from outside the TBS system. The legislation as applied to the psychopathic disorder sufferer in the UK is more complex as far as care and management in the health care sector are concerned.

Recent attempts to clarify the difficulties that clinicians experience during the course of their work when using UK law have met with despair and resignation. This is because amendments to the Mental Health Act 1983 (enacted by The Crime (Sentences) Act 1997) did not make the required changes to ensure that this group of patients received appropriate care (insufficient separation within legislation being made between the psychopathic and the mentally ill offender). This omission obscured the positive effects that legislative changes could have had for the psychopathic disordered patient as clinical staff concentrated on identifying the potential injustices of the new legislation for the mentally ill.

Implications for the care of the psychopathic individual

The treatment, care and management of the psychopathic disordered patient have raised moral dilemmas and will continue to do so. In the moral sense, the condition is different from any other mental disorder because of the very strong sense of selfishness: the sufferer perceives the rights of others to be of much lower importance than his or her own. Therefore, the sufferer has a tendency to use others as a means of achieving his or her ends, whether or not this involves the use of physical aggression in the process. There is also the lack of ability to make informed choices based on the considerations of all relevant options. This does not in any way suggest that psychopathic disordered individuals lack the capacity for understanding how to take advantage of social opportunities in a constructive way. On the contrary, they can (and at times do) contribute positively. However, a most significant factor in clinical diagnosis is the psychopath's willingness to take cruel advantage of others and the absence of any belief that it would be morally wrong to do so. Put simply, individuals with psychopathy do not appear to have an enduring understanding that, before they have their rights respected by others, they have the moral duty to respect the rights of others.

Further complicating the issue of treatment is the very unclear link between the mental health and offending behaviour of the person diagnosed as suffering from psychopathic disorder, so that the effectiveness of treatment is difficult to gauge. Current mental health services are not geared towards the effective satisfaction of the needs of this very volatile (but vulnerable) group of people. For example, the mix of various diagnostic groups in clinical areas does not lend itself to developing effective nursing skills to provide care for the needs of the patient. The focus on community care has made many psychiatric services concentrate on the care of the acutely ill patient. The very nature of the challenges posed by the psychopathic disordered patient means that the length of stay in hospital is longer than that for many other diagnostic groups. This scenario is more problematic to the medium secure units (MSUs), where levels of security are lower and facilities poorer, than to the high-security hospitals.

Another implication for treatment is the phenomenon of 'burn-out'. Proponents of this theory argue that psychopaths do eventually 'burn out'; that is, they suggest that there is a tendency for destructive behaviours to diminish at a certain age (arguably between the mid-20s and the mid-40s) (Curran and Partridge, 1963; Davis, 1967; Henderson and Batchelor, 1962). However, Walters (1990) shed more light on this phenomenon by attempting to separate burn-out from maturity, asserting in the process that 'criminal burn-out' does not imply maturity. It is clear, however, that the psychopath can mature after a certain age, a situation that can clearly be attributable to the realisation that the pleasure-seeking and self-serving ideologies of the youthful years are not a substitute for a lifestyle that includes developing longer-term relationships, clearer aspirations and a sense of responsibility. The question that remains concerns what do we do for these people in the interim. What is clearly required is the development of an urgent strategy for service provision taking into account the needs of the patient group, and that is why the recommendations of the Reed Review are timely. Its focus on the assessment of need and the clarification of treatment options should inform effective service planning in a more coherent fashion.

Treatment modalities for psychopathic disorder

The greatest determinant for restricting the liberty of the psychopathic disorder patient is the level of danger that he or she poses to others. The management of the individual therefore involves an assessment of the extant risks. The risk is normally assessed according to the particular circumstances of the individual, irrespective of the nature of the disorder. The difficulty of this approach, however, is that, although the patient can recall the circumstances surrounding the offence and is able to explain his or her thoughts and feelings – sometimes graphically – experience indicates that it is unwise to rely solely upon what is being said. Because of this, the outcomes of approaches to care may be unpredictable and unmeasurable as far as their being effective is concerned. Consequently, it has been argued that multiple treatment approaches should be employed in assisting the sufferer.

The difficulty of identifying a treatment that works is that very little information exists on the efficacy of treatments for this condition. In both the British and Dutch experiences, therapeutic communities are the only approach that has produced enough information that is worth replicating (Dolan and Coid, 1993). Other forms of treatment describe positive outcomes without adequately identifying what happens during the treatment process. The survey of nurses' views (Sallah, 1994) showed a great preference amongst nurses for cognitive behavioural therapies, dynamic psychotherapies and, in some cases, drug therapy.

Essential to the treatment of the patient group is the environment in which the person is to receive care. The survey of nurses' views showed that the most favoured initial placement for the sufferer was in an MSU with supporting services from community agencies through to high-security hospitals. Furthermore, nurses generally preferred a ward of patients with similar diagnoses to mixing various types of mental disorder, a preference not too dissimilar from the approach adopted in the Dutch TBS system.

Nursing psychopathic disorder patients

Contrary to the general view held by many, particularly those from other professional groups, nurses are, on the whole, pleased to work with psychopathic disorder patients. In the 1993 study referred to above, 86% ($n=80$) of respondents stated they would be happy to be involved in the care of the patient group if given the appropriate training. Those who were unwilling to be involved in working with the patient group expressed the view that, if attention were paid to the patient mix, they might reconsider their views. Others expressed the view that the care of the psychopathic disorder individual is too frustrating and unrewarding, as well as being laden with the risk of damaging inquiries when things go wrong. Public acceptance, and that of non-clinical staff, of the psychopath is without doubt of great relevance to the care of this group of people.

The Kirkman Inquiry (West Midlands Regional Health Authority, 1991) team, when addressing the problem posed by the individual throughout the rehabilitation process, observed that (for psychopathic disorder):

> there is widespread acceptance that there are no reliable objective or laboratory tests such as are available to colleagues in general medicine or forensic science.

To inform the process of risk assessment and to identify the degree of dangerousness, they suggested an amalgam of the following criteria:

- the past history of the patient;
- self-reporting by the patient at interview;
- observation by trained staff of both the behaviour and the mental state of the patient;
- discrepancies between what is reported and what is observed;
- some psychological tests, such as the polygraph and penile plethysmography;
- psychological testing, including inventory techniques for measuring personality traits and semantic differentials for shifts in conceptual thinking;
- statistics derived from studies of related cases, and prediction indicators derived from research.

What is patently obvious is the fact that no professional group has any monopoly over the determination and implementation of care for this group of patients. Psychologists see this as their domain and want clinical responsibility. This view was rejected by both nurses and consultant psychiatrists (Cope, 1993) consulted as part of the Reed Review. Nurses, however, have a significant role to play.

The survey of nurses' views in 1993 (Sallah, 1994) highlighted the view that the facilities currently available are inadequate. In terms of legislation, the majority of nurses are of the opinion that the present arrangements for the transfer of psychopathic disordered patients from prisons should be amended. This suggests a strong preference for a hybrid order to enable a more meaningful movement of patients between the prisons and NHS. This plea seems to have been listened to by Parliament (albeit in part) through the introduction of the changes to Section 38 of the Mental Health Act 1983. The survey also elicited the types of treatment approach that might be suitable. Cognitive behavioural approaches were generally favoured as the treatment of choice, followed by dynamic psychotherapy (although many thought that *milieu* psychotherapy might be useful).

Caring for the psychopathic disordered patient raises many issues, principally relating to treatability, boundaries, relationships and security. Storey and Dale (1998) examined reports that have highlighted these difficulties. Indeed, the governmental inquiry into the Personality Disorder Unit at Ashworth high-security hospital (the Committee of Inquiry chaired by Judge Fallon being due to report in early 1999) has reinforced the sense of urgency that some-thing must be done to develop a system that works. Storey and Dale have advanced the view that staff who work with this group of patients are experiencing problems in designing effective treatment packages, adopting the best way of dealing with issues of boundaries and relationships, and managing security.

In addressing some of these issues, Storey et al (1997) reported a collaboration between the High Security Psychiatric Services Commissioning Board, Ashworth Hospital Authority and the University of Central Lancashire, Preston, to develop a multidisciplinary framework of professional and vocational standards focused upon competency-based job descriptions and qualifications at a range of academic levels. This approach builds on that employed with social therapists (the Dutch TBS model) and a generic educational pathway to various professional groups (the British National Vocational Qualification movement). Other developments, for example the Risk Assessment, Management and Audit System

(RAMAS) developed by O'Rourke and colleagues, provide a basis for multidisciplinary approaches to identifying risk and formulating management strategies aiming to manage the problems identified (O'Rourke et al, 1997). Similarly, the work of Robinson et al (1996) has provided another dimension in the search for effective risk management packages to use in the care of the psychopathic disorder patient.

These initiatives, when seen in conjunction with the recent changes to the operation of the Mental Health Act 1983 – extensions of Section 38 (Interim Hospital Order) and changes to Sections 47 and 49 (transfer from prison to hospital) – have provided, and will continue to supply provide new ways of enabling practitioners, particularly nurses, to provide a better input to the care of this patient group.

The solutions to the problems posed by psychopathic disorder patients are receiving increased attention within the forensic services, and nurses are leading the way in the search for evidence to support effective methods of working. Nurses are taking lead roles in formulating care plans and are also able to evaluate their effectiveness when using the psychological therapies. What is required to enable effective management of the patient group is the cessation of the tendency of mixing various patient groups on the same ward. This is why the Reed Review recommendation for the establishment of assessment centres within the health and prison services is a step in the right direction. Multiprofessional and multiagency working will enrich the quality of the services offered to service users.

The preregistration training of nurses provides some understanding of the challenges that psychopathic disorder patients might present from the practical perspective. They are more able to understand the reasons behind patients' behaviours and are able to make effective contributions to care-planning. More and more nurses are being trained in advanced sociological and psychological therapies. The advent of the nurse practitioner and the work being done in nursing/practice development units has also demonstrated the nursing contribution to the care and management of this very difficult patient group.

Consistency in the *milieu* is important, particularly in conveying a caring, non-punitive and predictable environment. This approach is essential and poses a great challenge to nurses as the psychopathic disorder patient may have been conditioned by authority figures who have been inconsistent. They can therefore be distrustful and try to manipulate nurses into actions that may prove them to be unreliable (the nurse, in other words, becoming part of a self-fulfilling prophecy). It is important to maintain consistency as some patients may set up double-bind situations in order to depict nurses as uncaring and insincere. Successes, albeit small, will all contribute to the development of a therapeutic alliance that will set the stage for positive learning experiences and enable constructive change and growth.

Conclusions

The overwhelming view is that nurses are ready and willing to make a significant contribution to the care of the psychopathic disorder patient provided that a real effort is made to improve on the policy, strategy and national framework situation as it exists in the late 1990s. Education and training are key to this enthusiasm; what is needed is empowerment of nurses who are providing care for psychopathic disorder patients so that their confidence can enable proactive treatment, care and management.

References

American Psychiatric Association (1980) Diagnostic and Statistical Manual of Mental Disorders, 3rd Ed, Revised. Washington DC: APA.

Blackburn R (1986) Patterns of personality deviation among violent offenders: replication and extension of an empirical taxonomy. British Journal of Criminology 26: 254–69.

Checkley H (1976) The Mask of Sanity, 5th Edn. St Louis: CV Mosby.

Cope R (1993) A survey of forensic psychiatrists' views on psychopathic disorder. Journal of Forensic Psychiatry 4(2): 215–35.

Curran D, Partridge M (1963) Psychological Medicine, 5th Edn. London: ES Livingstone.

Davis DR (1967) Introduction to Psychopathology. Oxford: Oxford University Press.

Department of Health and Social Security (1986) Offenders suffering from psychopathic disorder (Health notice: HN(86)28). London: Department of Health and Social Security.

Department of Health and Home Office (1994) Review of Health and Social Services for Mentally Disordered Offenders and Others Requiring Similar Services (The Reed Review). Cmnd 2088. London: Department of Health and Home Office.

Dolan B, Coid J (1993) Psychopathic and Antisocial Personality Disorder, Treatment and Research Issues. London: Gaskell.

Fick (1947) Report of the Commission for the Further Extension of the Prison System. The Hague: Ministry of Justice.

Gunn J, Robertson G (1976) Psychopathic personality: a conceptual problem. Psychological Medicine 6: 631–4.

Hare RD (1991) The Hare Psychopathy Checklist – Revised. Toronto: Multi-Health Systems.

Henderson D, Batchelor I (1962) Henderson and Gillespie's Textbook of Psychiatry, 9th Edn. Oxford: Oxford University Press.

Home Office and Department of Health and Social Security (1975) Report of the

Committee on Mentally Abnormal Offenders (The Butler Report). London: HMSO.

O'Rourke MM, Hammond SM, Davies EJ (1997) Risk assessment and risk management – the way forward. Psychiatric Care 4(3): 104–6.

Robinson D, Reed V, Lange A (1996) Developing risk assessment scales in forensic psychiatric care. Psychiatric Care 3(4): 146–52.

Royal Commission (1957) The Royal Commission on the Law Relating to Mental Illness and Mental Deficiency (The Percy Report). London: HMSO.

Sallah D (1994) Views of the future care of psychopathic disordered patients. Psychiatric Care 2(4): 129–32.

Storey L, Dale C (1998) Meeting the needs of patients with severe personality disorders. Mental Health Practice 1(5): 20–6.

Storey L, Dale C, Martin E (1997) Social therapy: a developing model of care for people with personality disorders. NT Research 2(3): 210–18.

Walters GD (1990) The Criminal Lifestyle: Patterns of Serious Criminal Conduct. Newbury Park, CA: Sage.

West Midlands Regional Health Authority (1991) Report of the Panel of Inquiry Appointed by the West Midlands Regional Health Authority and the Special Hospitals Service Authority To Investigate the Case of Kim Kirkman. Birmingham: West Midlands RHA.

Chapter 4
Diverting people with mental health problems from the criminal justice system

GINA HILLIS

All those whose mental health problems culminate in their becoming entangled in the criminal justice system should, as a matter of principle, be diverted into the appropriate health care services. Where this is not possible, there should be provision for appropriate mental health care within police custody and during the transition between court and prison, whether they be remanded or convicted. Apart from the obvious duty of psychiatric agencies to ensure that this service is provided, it is economical in financial and human terms for both the individual and the community in general to divert appropriate individuals from custody.

The beginnings of enlightenment

The Home Office Circular *Provision for Mentally Disordered Offenders* (Home Office, 1990a) identified the urgent need for mental health care services to be established within the criminal justice system and recommended a complete review of the situation in order to implement radical changes. This Circular stated that 'a mentally disordered person should never be remanded to prison simply to receive medical treatment or assessment'. The Reed Review (Department of Health and Home Office, 1992) indicated that there should be collaboration between all the agencies involved in the care of MDOs and those with similar needs, and laid down guidelines to facilitate co-operation. Both the Circular and the Reed Review considered the possibilities of early intervention and diversion where appropriate as a preventive measure against the deterioration of MDOs while in custody.

Tumin (Home Office, 1990b) had indicated the problems and extent of suicidal and self-harming behaviours within prisons, and a further report by Tumin and Woolf (Home Office, 1991), which examined the causes of a series of prison disturbances, demonstrated the very unsatisfactory nature of prisons for inmates, well and unwell alike. This report indicated that significant changes to both the environment and regimes of control and care were necessary as a matter of urgency. The effects were to raise the general awareness of the plight of inmates and MDOs within penal institutions, create a more humanistic paradigm in some echelons of the criminal justice system and give a political edge to the neglected area of penal reform. This enabled opportunities for changes in service provision to be planned as funding for new initiatives became accessible. A sense of motivation and a 'can do' feel began to emerge among the forensic clinical professionals who provide care and treatment for MDOs as it appeared that health care within the criminal justice system, and prisons in particular, began to take the first steps towards considering and adopting NHS paradigms of care and treatment. An age of enlightment within the criminal justice system had commenced.

Diversion from custody

There was much debate in the late 1980s and early 1990s about the concept and definition of diversion from custody. McKittrick and Eysenck (1984) defined it as 'the halting or suspending of proceedings against an accused person in favour of processing through a non-criminal disposition'. The term 'diversion service' offers fuller meaning in that an accused person is provided with an alternative service or at least extra ways in which to receive the mental health and psychiatric care that he or she requires. This may entail straight diversion from custody and prosecution, or the appropriate psychiatric care and treatment in tandem with the legal process. As in the general population, individuals with mental health problems find themselves in contact with the criminal justice system – some through no direct fault of their own – as bewildered parties to events or as the victims or perpetrators of crime. Diversion from custody services is focused upon the needs of those who fall into the latter category.

The UK had approximately 60 diversion schemes in operation in 1994 (Backer-Holst, 1994). However, this figure was subject to the vagaries of definition, and several schemes were funded for a 'pump-priming' period of time (usually up to 3 years) but were unable to attract further funding when this period of time elapsed.

There are now over 100 schemes in the UK at various stages of development that interact with a variety of points within the criminal justice system. Similar services are to be found in other parts of the developed world, including Australia, New Zealand and the USA.

The nature of the diversion scheme depends largely upon local determining factors, including the maturity of interagency relationships and collaborative intent; demographic factors such as the characteristics of the the population (health, unemployment and poverty); social support structures; criminological characteristics of the local population; the density of criminal justice system provision in the area; and the availability of NHS mental health acute, intensive care, high-dependency and medium secure mental health facilities. Different forms of provision are required for highly populated cities, with multiple police stations feeding into busy central courts, whilst those needed within rural areas involve smaller police stations and courts sitting for only a few sessions each week. A tailor-made approach is required for each area, and some have developed on-call services, with a nurse or psychiatrist serving one or more police stations and often one or more courts. These schemes offer a visiting service to assess at a designated time each week those persons thought to have a mental health problem.

Many offer an emergency service as well as providing regular input. Other schemes have set up panel assessment teams, which are multiagency and take referrals from the courts as well as providing assessment and diversion. These schemes tend to be reactive. Follow-up care is often provided in addition. Suffice it to say that all schemes and established services operate differently and are currently undergoing a period of rapid development. Some of the busier city area schemes provide a daily service to the main courts, the prison and the police stations and have a proactive approach.

Interagency liaison and collaboration

Some regions of the country have developed integrated local Diversion from Custody Panels, which liaise regularly or can be called into session at short notice to ensure that appropriate support is mobilised. For example, in the Greater Manchester area, there are 10 Diversion from Custody Panels consisting of representatives from the police, probation, social services, housing and the NHS – the latter usually a CPN. All have access to expert forensic psychiatric medical, nursing and social work expert advice, and the

Crown Prosecution Service (CPS) is engaged as necessary. An overview of trends is maintained by the Greater Manchester MDO Services Co-ordinating Group. This is a county-wide group with senior representation from all the aforementioned agencies plus standing members from the NHS Regional Office, the CPS and the Courts (GMMDOCG, 1996). Members of this regional group are of sufficient seniority to make things happen, quickly, should that be necessary.

The key elements in a comprehensive approach to diversion working include the creation and maintenance of efficient and good-natured liaison between the wide range of agencies and disciplines who all have a legitimate part to play in creating a web of care for vulnerable individuals. In our experience, effective diversion schemes are worked by those who feel confident enough to say that they have not got an answer, as is much informal networking concerning individual cases. There is also a clear understanding of the opportunities afforded by joint working, in addition to an acknowledgement of some of the limitations; for example, ask anyone working in a diversion scheme about some of the issues that regularly occur around confidentiality of information. Also, of course, everyone remains painfully aware that a few mentally disordered persons will seek to get through the web of support as they perceive it to be a keep-net.

Diversion may occur at several junctures of the criminal justice system, including:

- at the point of arrest (the police);
- from the judiciary (the courts);
- from remand (the prisons) or conviction (the prisons or probation).

Contact at the point of arrest

Contact with the NHS diversion from custody system occasionally occurs when those in police custody are taken to accident and emergency departments where persons with expertise (usually mental health nurses) are employed or where a referral is made by the accident and emergency staff to a duty psychiatrist for an urgent opinion. However, the most common stage at which contact with diversion services is likely is at the point of arrest, when a person is conveyed from an incident to the police station for questioning (Table 4.1).

Table 4.1. Potential opportunities for diversion from custody

Criminal justice system agency	Point of contact
Police custody:	Point of arrest At an NHS accident and emergency department Police cells – referral by custody sergeant or police surgeon
Court custody	Custody Referral by the Clerk of the Court Court clinics Remand to hospital for assessment/treatment
Prisons custody	Psychiatric emergency while in prison Request for assessment while on remand Request for assessment while serving a sentence Prison clinics Therapies delivered by NHS personnel in prisons
Probation	Referral by Court Probation Officer Bail hostel

Being arrested is an extremely traumatic and testing time for a healthy person, but for a person with a mental health problem, it is likely to be even more confusing and frightening. The need for experienced mental health professionals to be actively involved in this process is not in doubt. Indeed, it would now be viewed as unorthodox for the NHS and criminal justice systems not to synchronise their activities in response to the needs of a vulnerable person who comes into contact with the law. In addition, the Police and Criminal Evidence Act 1984 requires the police to ensure that certain vulnerable individuals (for example, minors and persons with some types of learning disability) have appropriate representation during questioning, and some NHS facilities now offer clinics and crisis support to police detention centres so that custody sergeants and police surgeons or forensic medical examiners can call for an opinion at any time while the person is in police custody.

Contact at the judiciary

Joseph (1992) observed the 'yawning gap' between the possible diversion of the mentally disordered person from the police station and the next available opportunity during remand in custody; diversion prior to or at the point of appearance in court affords an opportunity to fill that yawning gap.

Awaiting a court appearance while in custody provokes significant levels of anxiety and increased levels of distress. The mentally disordered individual requires sensitive and tactful support and interventions at this time; the level of competence required is that of a mature and experienced health and/or social care practitioner. This is necessary to ensure that the person optimises his or her mental health strengths at this time in order to be best placed to face the ordeal ahead. In this environment, the clinical professional requires a sophisticated understanding of the machinations of the criminal justice system, insight into the possible options for disposal by the court and knowledge of the ability of the local health care facilities to be able to support the individual who is in custody. Diversion schemes in these environments range from regular court clinic arrangements run by psychiatrists and visits to the holding cells by CPNs prior to courts commencing each day, to responses to emergency calls from the Clerk of the Court for advice and/or assessment on request of the magistrates, to be carried out prior to an individual's reappearing before them later the same day.

Contact after remand

Custodial remand offers a further stage at which diversion from custody may be considered. There are a number of people with mental health problems who are inappropriately remanded into prison (or to bail hostels) because their vulnerabilities have not been recognised. Others are remanded into custody in spite of earlier attempts at diversion – this situation may occur for a number of reasons, most commonly because an appropriate health care option is unavailable or the gravity of the offence with which the person is charged does not allow diversion to take place at an earlier stage because of public interest considerations. Inmates of prisons (convicts) and residents of probation hostels may also be referred for assessment and possible mental health interventions.

Various models of NHS input have developed with regard to the prisons, and these are, to some extent, determined by the gaps in the skills of the staff in the prison health care centres (some of whom are highly competent in managing difficult inmates). Many diversion schemes at this point, in the first instance, originate as psychiatric clinics run by health professionals in the health care centre. For prisoners, this is rather like booking in to see a general practitioner (although it is usual for the prison medical officer to screen individuals asking for assistance). Available are clinics and health check visits to the landings and wings by NHS personnel, therapeutic input on a needs basis and, if necessary, relocation to NHS facilities to give therapy that cannot be successfully undertaken within the prison environment. For example, the Adolescent and Adult Forensic Services at Salford, near Manchester, have a variety of inputs to several local prisons, including HMPs Hindley, Manchester, Risley and Styal. These inputs are delivered by forensic psychiatrists, clinical nurse specialists and occupational therapists. A community sex offender treatment programme offers an additional option for diverting offenders from custody, utilising Probation Orders. At Parc Prison in South Wales, the NHS South Wales Forensic Psychiatric Service provides a total health care package for all the inmates – from general health care through to forensic psychiatric input. This unique arrangement offers possibilities for the most responsive form of diversion scheme for the prison service, although it is yet too early to make meaningful comparisons with other models of input.

Case study: the city of Birmingham

Birmingham, a city and conurbation in the West Midlands, has a population of approximately 2,146,000. The city has a wide representation of persons from differing social classes and ethnic and cultural backgrounds. Like any metropolis, it has its share of deprived areas and centres of high unemployment, with all their associated problems, as well as areas of relative wealth.

Diversion at the point of arrest: the DAPA scheme

There are 12 main police stations in the Birmingham conurbation. One of these, in South Birmingham, was selected to pilot a diversion at the point of arrest scheme (DAPA; Wix, 1993) for 1 year, commencing in 1992. A forensic CPN (FCPN) from Reaside Clinic (the South Birmingham forensic psychiatric MSU) visited the station cells on a daily basis in order to screen all those arrested to ascertain their mental health status. It quickly became apparent that many arrests occurred during the late evening and throughout the night, and the MSU responded by providing an additional on-call service. This service has been in operation for 6 years and has been extended to service the requirements of five police stations in the city of Birmingham.

The first year of the DAPA scheme provided an opportunity for the police to become familiar with the recognition of mental health problems and the process of diversion at the point of arrest. Over

700 people were screened and assessed, 7% of whom were found to have a mental health problem; 50% of these were diverted at this point. Most required further assessment and treatment in the community, but some required admission to the local psychiatric hospital. The majority of the 7% were not charged following successful arrangements for diversion, but a small number could not be diverted and were required to appear before the magistrates in view of the seriousness of their offences.

Diversion from the judiciary – at the Magistrates' Court

Birmingham Magistrates' Court is a large complex of 24 courts situated in the city centre. Each day, all the surrounding police stations feed remanded persons into the central custody cells. Under the Magistrates' Court Act 1980, a defendant must be brought to the next available court (usually within 24 hours). The courts sit every day except Sundays, Good Friday and Christmas Day. On each working day, a court processes all those who have been arrested within the preceding 24 hours.

The diversion service in the Magistrates' Court commenced as a pilot scheme at the beginning of 1991, and early results demonstrated the need for such a service. It now forms an integral part of the Birmingham diversion services. The main aim is to provide a proactive approach to screening and identifying mental health problems in the court custody population. Proactivity is a much more rewarding method of working rather than adopting a reactive role of waiting for referrals from others (Hillis, 1993).

An FCPN from the MSU commences work very early each court day in order to screen the prosecution files and assess prior to their court appearances those defendants who are thought to have mental health problems. It is common to have 25 defendants, who have been remanded overnight, of whom three are likely to show some indication of being potentially vulnerable as the result of a possible mental disorder. These individuals are screened in more depth using specific assessment criteria.

The role of the FCPN: assessment

Our experience is that FCPNs are best placed to undertake this role as:

* they are skilled in mental health screening (Rooney and Tarbuck, 1997);

- they are aware of the local NHS facilities should they be required;
- they have insight as a result of their forensic service experience into what forms of disposal might be appropriate for individuals (and can therefore help the individual to prepare for what might happen);
- they are more flexible than other colleagues (because of their willingness to be stretched and because of their strength in numbers, which enables the workforce to be malleable) in being able rapidly to respond to requests for assistance;
- because they are nurses, with a popular acceptance by the public and good training, they are able rapidly to befriend individuals and impart a caring approach in extremely trying cirumstances.

The value system of the nurse, as of other health care professionals, should ensure that the defendant's encounter with the diversion scheme is free of pejorative or punitive overtones: the nurse is there to support and care as well as to assess.

Assessments are preceded by an explanation to the defendant, who is given the choice not to be assessed. In practice, refusal to co-operate is rare. The issue of guilt or innocence has no relevance to the assessment, the focus being upon the mental health of the individual and assisting in relieving the distress caused by the individual's predicament, which may be exacerbating an existing mental illness. The boundaries of confidentiality are explained to the defendant. The nurses' *Code of Professional Conduct* (UKCC, 1993), along with its subsidiary publications and the South Birmingham Mental Health Services NHS Trust Procedures, is used to reinforce the nature of the confidential relationship. The assessment interview is semi-structured and involves data collection sufficient to establish whether indicators of mental health problems or of mental disorder are present. During the first 5 years of this scheme, 51% of those assessed using this method have had an identified mental health problem or mental disorder that has led to recommendations being made to the magistrate.

When an identified mental health problem is established, further in-depth assessment is indicated. The FCPN will seek to examine in detail issues such as past history, precipitators of presenting behaviour, social support networks, the abuse of illicit substances and alcohol abuse. He or she will assess the defendant's mood, cognitive functioning and thought content, perceptual experiences and level of understanding. The reaction to the present situation also provides indicators of the mental health of the individual. Factors such as age, gender, physical health and current prescribed medication are considered, as are recent changes in sleep, appetite and lifestyle. Commonly presenting psychiatric phenomena include thought disorders and/or delusional or hallucinatory experiences, including ideas of reference, grandiose ideas, beliefs of being controlled by others or reports of unusual and bizarre experiences.

Risk assessment

Particular attention is paid to risk factors associated with past thoughts of, or attempts at, suicide, indicators of past or present self-harming behaviours or thoughts, and contemporary parasuicidal ideas: any evidence of planning suicide or self-harm in the recent past indicates that the defendant is vulnerable and is at serious and high risk. The FCPNs are required to judge the effects of the feelings associated with being remanded in custody and appearing before magistrates, including anger at oneself, anger at others, shame and guilt as these may lead the defendant to have a reduced locus of internal control, impulsive acts becoming more probable under these conditions.

The assessment attempts to define a collection of presenting indications of mental health and ill-health so that a nursing diagnosis may be made and an accurate report based on observations given to a psychiatrist should that be necessary. A dilemma for the nurse when reporting findings to magistrates is that the FCPN is experientially competent to provisionally diagnose serious mental illnesses (and others), although he or she has no legal competence to do so; thus, the nurse must be careful about how reports are imparted. All assessments are documented and remain confidential. A brief written résumé of findings is made available to others with a bona fide interest in the defendant, and verbal interactions take place with those who are appropriately involved, such as the Crown Prosecution Service (CPS) and Court Probation Officer, in order to suggest an appropriate way to proceed. Given that Magistrates' Courts are public places (as they have public and press galleries), utmost discretion is required in report-giving in order to avoid breaching the defendant's confidence. Section 23(3) of the Prosecution of Offences Act 1985 allows a prosecuting officer to discontinue a case if it is felt to be in the interests of the defendant not to continue, and not in the public interest to proceed, provided that appropriate care is arranged.

Information obtained from a defendant during assessment may be of a sensitive nature: an admission of other criminal activities, threatening suicide or incriminating evidence (about self or others).

In these circumstances, the FCPN consults medical colleagues at the MSU on the ethical issues associated with the possession of such information in relation to the defendant's confidentiality and the safety of the defendant and others. In practice, this has been a rare occurrence.

During the first 5 years of operation, over 2500 people were assessed while they were defendants at court, and just over 50% were found to have a mental health problem. Approximately 20% of these required admission to hospital by either informal or compulsory means, Sections 2 or 3 of the Mental Health Act 1983 being used to effect compulsory admissions to hospital. Over 60% required outpatient treatment or follow-up in the community, the remainder needing admission to the MSU for learning disabilities or, in the case of dangerous offending behaviour, urgent psychiatric assessments at the health care centre during first remand into custody in prison. The ratio of females to males being assessed was 1:9. The ethnic breakdown of those assessed showed an overrepresentation of African Caribbean and Asian people compared with the number in the general population of Birmingham.

There were occasions when diversion was not successful at this point, usually because of a lack of hospital beds, disputes over catchment areas (particularly if the defendant was of no fixed abode) or the inability to find suitable accommodation for bail purposes. Bail is often denied if there is a lack of community ties or if the defendant is of no fixed abode and is thought likely to abscond and not reappear. The law regarding bail is laid down in the Bail Act 1976.

Diversion schemes and the prisons

Some defendants, for whom earlier attempts at diversion were unsuccessful, are remanded into custody, initially for a 7 day period, and still require psychiatric treatment. A forensic nurse from the MSU visits Birmingham prison each day to screen and assess all prisoners received within the previous 24 hours. These prisoners come not only from Birmingham courts, but also from other surrounding courts, and all are filtered by the screening nurse. The same assessment procedure takes place and the health care centre is used when a prisoner is found to have a mental health problem or mental illness. Following discussion with staff in the centre, the visiting psychiatrist is requested to assess the prisoner with a view to hospital admission to local hospitals or medium secure facilities. This service has been operational since March 1993 and is now integral to the diversion scheme. The population of Birmingham prison is male, and there is as yet no such diversion service for females, many of whom are remanded to prisons outside the West Midlands.

During the first 2 years of this prison diversion scheme, 1700 newly remanded prisoners were assessed, of whom just under 50% had a mental health problem, 25% of these requiring immediate admission to the health care centre. The remaining 75% required various interventions, for example recommendations to reside in a multicell as suicidal views had been expressed. Others were referred to drug or alcohol treatment groups and anxiety management groups. Some were referred to the prison health care nurses who visit the prison wings and landings in a similar way to the FCPNs visiting in the community. Diversion from prison was achieved for 3.5% of prisoners, some of whom were bailed on second court appearance and some of whom were admitted to hospitals using Sections 47 and 48 of the Mental Health Act 1983. The service was quickly extended to assess sentenced prisoners and those subject to deportation proceedings.

Follow-up of divertees in the community

Another aspect of the role of the FCPN in the diversion scheme is short-term community follow-up for those persons diverted from prison or not disposed of with a custodial sentence who require psychiatric care but for whom links have not yet been forged with local services. The FCPN ensures that breakdowns in communication do not occur at this vulnerable juncture, and the FCPN maintains contact with all the agencies relevant to the individual until a satisfactory care package is in place, which may entail the FCPN offering support to other agencies until they feel comfortable working with the individual concerned. This caseload also contains divertees from other stages of the DAPA scheme: police stations and courts. The time between the first involvement of the FCPN on a community basis and the transfer of involvement with the individual to local services is generally 2–4 months.

Some community follow-up work involves visiting local bail hostels, and one particular hostel in Birmingham city specialises in providing for MDOs. The role of the FCPN includes offering support and advice to this hostel, which was the first of its kind, opened in 1993. The aim of the hostel is to compile a package of care and provision by assessing the mental state of its residents, and then to work in close liaision with the Bail Information Service to ensure that good advice is offered to the courts.

Training for the future

The DAPA scheme was developed on the basis of developing awareness, insight and understanding between agencies and across
systems. This included regular and *ad hoc* meetings, joint training
events and staff secondments and exchanges. Nationally, various
forms of training were developed, also on an *ad hoc* basis in order to
inform practitioners of what to expect of diversion schemes and of
other agencies.

In Birmingham, the MSU decided to invest heavily in training for
the future by developing a training course for which approval was
sought from the ENB. Approval was given to run an accredited
course at certificate level. The courses completed so far have been
modular, based on a mix of academic input and competency demonstration in the workplace, and are offered on a part-time basis (day
and block release) over 6 months. Early students completing the
course feel that their abilities have been enhanced, but research is
required to demonstrate the benefits of having attended the course.

Conclusions

The number of diversion from custody schemes has grown dramati-
cally in the 1990s, and diversion from custody is viewed as an
enlightened mental health practice. The nature of the schemes varies
significantly from area to area. The DAPA scheme in Birmingham
has been described in order to illustrate the various levels at which
diversion from custody may occur.

A number of agencies and professional disciplines are involved in
providing successful diversion from custody schemes, and indeed,
without co-operation based upon a common understanding, aims
and goodwill diversion schemes will fail. The process of developing
DAPA and other diversion from custody schemes requires sustained
effort in the form of liaison, joint training and staff exchanges.
There are differing and legitimate opinions on which agency and
profession should take the lead in this form of service provision.
FCPNs are ideally placed to lead most schemes because of their
training, skills base and relative versatility. They are also in a good
position to befriend individuals in circumstances in which the
person's liberty may be threatened by contact with other agencies
and disciplines. Additionally, the FCPN is uniquely placed to co-
ordinate health care packages that span the criminal justice system
and NHS provision.

Diversion from custody offers the potential to relieve the criminal justice system of the pressures associated with attempting to care for mentally ill persons within a system that is likely to reinforce aspects of the mental disorder or exacerbate existing conditions. Staff members within the system are often pleased to know that NHS professionals are available to offer support, advice and assistance. The cost benefit of schemes such as the Birmingham DAPA has not yet been researched, but those involved confidently predict that the savings to the criminal justice system will be substantial. The cost of treating the ill defendant, or the MDO, is more likely to be borne by the relevant health authority, which is appropriate.

The vulnerable person caught up in the criminal justice system is bewildered and frightened. Some such individuals are incapable of exercising their legal rights, and some celebrated miscarriages of justice have indeed occurred because of this. From the individual's perspective, he or she retains the right to receive appropriate health care when it is required, whether this be in liberty or in custody. The need for a proactive service is necessary in this respect, and diversion schemes form part of this proactive response from society to care for its most vulnerable. Prior to the DAPA scheme in Birmingham, and diversion from custody schemes in general, screening of the vulnerable was left to those not employed for this purpose, who were without the necessary skills to detect signs of mental ill health. Multiagency risk panels, District Diversion Panels as in Manchester, and comprehensive approaches to diversion from custody as in Birmingham, may help to ensure that some of the tragedies that have occurred in the community – wherein MDOs have assaulted or killed others – are less likely to occur as a communication and support matrix exists to provide care for those who appear on the local supervision register.

References

Backer-Holst A (1994) A new window of opportunity. Psychiatric Care (Mar/Apr): 15–18.

Department of Health and Home Office (1992) Review of Health and Social Services for Mentally Disordered Offenders and Others Requiring Similar Services (The Reed Review). Cmnd 2088. London: HMSO.

GMMDOCG (Greater Manchester Mentally Disordered Offender Co-ordinating Group) (1996) Responding to the Needs of the Mentally Disordered Offender and Others with Similar Needs: Report of the MDO Steering Groups in Greater Manchester. Warrington: NHS Executive Regional Office.

Hillis G (1993) Diverting tactics. Nursing Times 89(1): 24.

Home Office (1990a) Provision for Mentally Disordered Offenders. HO Circular 66/90. London: HMSO.

Home Office (1990b) Report on a Review by Her Majesty's Chief Inspector of Prisons –
    Suicide and Self Harm in the Prison Service Establishments in England and Wales
    (The Tumin Report). Cmnd 1383. London: HMSO.
Home Office (1991) Report on Prison Disturbances – April 1990 (The Woolf Report).
    Cmnd 1456. London: HMSO.
Joseph PL (1992) Mentally disordered homeless offenders: diversion from custody.
    Health Trends 22(2): 51–3.
McKittrick N, Eysenck S (1984) Diversion – a bit fix. Justice of the Peace (16 Jun): 337.
Rooney J, Tarbuck P (1997) Buying Forensic Mental Health Nursing: An RCN Guide
    for Purchasers. London: RCN.
UKCC (United Kingdom Central Council for Nursing, Midwifery and Health Visiting)
    (1993) Code of Professional Conduct, 3rd Edn. London: UKCC.
Wix S (1993) Diversion at the point of arrest. Psychiatric Care (Jul/Aug): 102–4.

Chapter 5
Forensic community mental health nurses and their self-perceived roles

MARIE TOMAN

This chapter concerns the results of a small-scale research exercise undertaken to explore the self-perceived roles of forensic community mental health nurses (FCMHNs). The original study was based on a total of 12 community nurses: 6 FCMHNs and 6 generic CPNs. For the purpose of this chapter, the focus will be on the outcomes for the FCMHNs, four of whom were male. The FCMHNs operated within and served a large geographical area, the individual nurse being responsible for that area of catchment.

Forensic community mental health nursing is a relatively young specialism of both forensic mental health nursing and community mental health nursing. There is much perceived overlap between the roles of the community mental health nurse (CMHN) and the FCMHN. Although it is not possible to claim that the findings from the research can be applied to all situations in which both CMHNs and FCMHNs practise, it is safe to make some generalisations, whilst also noting that the six FCMHNs used in the sample were drawn from services with consolidated experience bases and recognised as centres of excellence by many statutory bodies, professional groups and external agencies.

Method

The six FCMHNs were interviewed. Discussion was centred around the practitioner's first interview with the patient and what it was hoped would be achieved. Data were collected through a semi-structured, open-ended interview schedule, were fully recorded and were transcribed for analysis in a qualitative manner. The approach to the analysis of the data was through a method described as 'content analy-

51

sis'. From the data, six main categories emerged: role, assessment, interpersonal skills, personal and work experience, self-presentation and training needs. Self-presentation emerged from generic CPN data only (so is not treated separately in this report), and the training needs identified as an adjunct to this study are briefly discussed.

Role of the FCMHN

FCMHNs worked flexible hours, with an average caseload of 15 clients, working half a week in the community and the remaining time in the court. In addition, they assist the multiprofessional team in operating a 24 hour on-call emergency service and 'open door' system. Flexible hours provided FCMHNs with a degree of autonomy in the way in which they worked and maintained contact with patients who would otherwise 'slip through the net'. Autonomy within the role assisted in reducing stress levels and was described as such by the majority of the respondents.

In addition to assessment, normalisation was achieved on occasions by meeting with and partnering patients in community activities, the primary aim being one of socialising. The decision would be self-initiated or in direct response to patient request. FCMHNs felt that this arrangement ensured some social contact where the patient was socially isolated and was considered by some respondents to be preferable to socialising in the patient's home and/or in day centres for the mentally ill. Some examples of the venues selected were cafés, pubs and restaurants. Admirably, where patient budgets were limited, respondents paid out of their own pockets.

The ongoing assessment of a patient's mental health, supervision, the restrictions imposed on his or her movement by conditions of discharge, and administering and monitoring medication, presented the FCMHN with a difficult balancing act between caring and fulfilling the requirements of the Mental Health Act 1983 and other statutes. Patients suffering from severe side-effects of neuroleptic drugs (which may for some patients be less tolerable than the actual illness) were described by FCMHNs and gave rise to dilemmas in practice, that is, in maintaining the patient's mental health and the subsequent safety of all. Overdependence on the use of neuroleptic drugs as a form of treatment has revealed dire consequences for many users. Irreversible side-effects are experienced by between one- and two-thirds of users, along with not-infrequent reports of sudden death. Mental health professionals must clearly develop and implement alternative approaches to managing psychosis.

User participation in service delivery

Care for people with severe mental health problems must be founded on services that are appropriate and acceptable to the patient group (Department of Health, 1994). NHS reforms and the movement towards the empowerment of patients have created a platform from which users can voice their views; their participation is an established feature of enlightened mental health services. However, it is noted that not all mental health workers are committed to user involvement (Campbell and Lindow, 1997). Quality service development is therefore dependent on collaboration between users, nurses and other professionals. Commissioning health authorities will also influence future service developments and will purchase health services based on specifications that state minimum quality and service requirements. An example of what service commissioners may expect of FCMHNs is indicated by the Royal College of Nursing guide to buying forensic mental health nursing (Rooney and Tarbuck, 1997; Figure 5.1).

Assessment

The assessment of mental health and subsequent risk was considered by all FCMHNs to be the major goal to be achieved at first interview, irrespective of the nature of the referral; it is also an ongoing process throughout patient care. Extreme contrasts in assessment working patterns were found, ranging from the use of no formal tools to the use

- Effective communication between forensic, generic and other agencies
- Assessment of the client and, if appropriate, his or her family
- Predischarge assessment and care-planning of the client prior to his or her return to the community, including detailed risk assessment
- Aftercare for those discharged from secure services
- An intensive level of skilled supervision
- A high level of responsibility and discretion to co-ordinate care, reduce risk and prevent relapse
- Advocacy on behalf of the client whose past behaviour has rendered him or her unpopular in the community
- Ongoing liaison between the health, social and probation services
- Involvement with court diversion schemes
- Assessment of people held in police custody
- Crisis intervention and management services
- Provision of advice and support to colleagues within generic services

Figure 5.1. Skills required of forensic community mental health nurses (After Rooney and Tarbuck, 1997.)

of standard instruments. Recording and reporting are, however, fundamental to effective care and risk management, and nurses failing to use systematic approaches to assessment are clearly failing to uphold their Code of Professional Conduct (UKCC, 1993). The consequences of inappropriate and non-recording have known risks associated with homicide and suicide by the mentally disordered (Boyd, 1996), and these risks are unacceptable bearing in mind the FCMHN's role in protecting both the patient and the public. Diagnosis and prediction are dependent upon the equitable, accurate and systematic reporting of disruptive behaviour on the part of the patient and – where relevant – the responses of significant others, so that a whole picture emerges.

Interprofessional co-operation was identified and described by FCMHNs as being crucial to quality care (Horder, 1992) yet is perceived to be rarely achieved. A radical structural change to further promote interagency working between mental health and social care services will hopefully bring about a change in service provision (Department of Health, 1997). FCMHNs experienced emotional effects and feelings of pressure, which had interfered in efficient and effective decision-making within the assessment process; respondents related this to their own inexperience of working in the community and, in particular, the courts. These factors indicated the importance of clinical supervision both to assist personal growth and to protect the client from practitioner fatigue.

Risk assessment

A number of FCMHNs were not confident in their ability to assess risk. The literature reflects this view and indicates that mental health clinicians – regardless of discipline – are poor at predicting risk. Much literature attempts to predict the risk associated with mental illness and subsequent crime (Cocozza and Steadman, 1974; Loucas, 1982; Prins, 1990; Scott, 1977; Steadman et al, 1978). Our understanding of violent behaviour, and instruments to predict its occurrence, is not sufficiently developed, so our understanding of the dynamics of violent behaviour is, at times, limited. Monahan (1988) indicated that:

- there were several major problems associated with assessing risk accurately, including instruments for measuring violence and predictions that were not sufficiently robust;
- research efforts were fragmented and lacked co-ordination;
- patient samples lacked breadth.

However, in acknowledging these limitations, accurate prediction, it is claimed, requires a number of research-based questions to be asked and defensibly substantiated so that a baseline can be formed against which judgements about risk may be tested (Crichton, 1995; Monahan, 1981, 1988; Pollock et al, 1989). The way forward is in placing more emphasis on assessment than prediction, with research that begins to describe and develop cogent and systematic approaches to clinical decision-making.

Interpersonal skills

The interpersonal qualities that were identified by the study – warmth, genuineness, empathy, respect, accepting, being a friend, treating a person as an equal, caring and self-awareness – are also identified by Rogers (1957) and are considered essential to developing a person-centred relationship and for bringing about a positive outcome for patients. Such qualities must be inherent within the therapist's value system and attitudes as Rogers goes on to suggest that they cannot be taught. Knowledge of the patient, his illness and the offence behaviour was described by the majority of respondents as having the potential to threaten them personally. Nevertheless, empathy, respect and a non-judgemental approach were factors to be achieved in a successful working relationship with patients.

The skills indicated by respondents to fulfil their roles could be mapped into Heron's (1975) conceptual framework of Six Category Intervention Analysis. As a method of identifying which interpersonal skills (and styles of interacting) are in use, Heron's model is potent and can assist individuals to address both balance and purpose in interactions. 'Counselling' was a term used to describe what occurred in practice and was identified as a skill requirement by some respondents. Interestingly, two FCMHNs did not perceive themselves as counsellors as they had not attended a counselling course. Listening and distracting skills were used regularly as necessary, and FCMHNs indicated that a 'non-display' of stress was a useful strategy to diffuse and deal with aggressive and difficult situations. Respondents also identified that these skills took time to develop. This confirms research findings that experienced staff are less likely to be assaulted than the inexperienced, with the helper who retains positive and productive thought processes gaining control of the situation more readily (Davies and Burgess, 1988; Howells and Hollin, 1989).

Interventions based on intuition were identified by respondents; these are viewed by some nursing theorists as evidence of inductive thought and grounding in experience (Chinn and Jacobs, 1991; Robinson and Vaughan, 1992). It is further suggested that, for some, this tacit knowledge is gained over time, practitioners expressing difficulties in verbalising their growing abilities along the route. Such approaches suggest that knowledge gained by experience is a 'ways of knowing' and suggests that openness to this, as well as to other more traditional ways of learning, is important in the development of nursing knowledge.

Personal and work experience

Life experience taken with reflection on nursing practice resulted in skill and knowledge acquisition for some respondents. With nursing knowledge embedded in practice itself, knowing and reflection, it is claimed, play a major part in skill acquisition and proficiency (Benner, 1984; Chinn and Jacobs, 1991). In addition, unconscious learning through subliminal perception adds to the overall experience and performance. Some FCMHNs described learning as having occurred through 'trial and error', not only appearing to view this as acceptable, but also incorporating specific interventions into their practice based on their own biases and beliefs (without apparent grounds). As the recipients of 'trial and error' practice, patients are exposed to an obvious risk of harm. This form of nurse practice does not comply with the UKCC Code of Professional Conduct (UKCC, 1993) and is therefore unacceptable. However, if a nurse does not have a theoretical base or conceptual framework on which to base his or her interventions, a reliance upon trial and error is inevitable. It further demonstrates an urgent need to generate a reliable knowledge of mental health care and validate practices based upon this knowledge.

Working in the 'front line' with patients, particularly patients presenting with extremely difficult management problems, can and does generate feelings of distress. There is a potential risk of nurses not feeling able to listen or not asking difficult questions because they fear that the content of any self-disclosures may have a possible impact on the nurse–patient relationship and consequently be counterproductive and interfere with the ongoing assessment. The failure to manage such stress could lead to life-threatening situations for the patient, nurse or significant others.

Working in the courts also presented difficulties. Here, FCMHNs indicated that the 'freshness' of the offence adversely affected their emotions. Some indicated that it took them a year to adjust to assimilating such knowledge without feeling threatened. There is an obvious area here for staff training in the management of anxiety.

Self-awareness and clinical supervision are considered central to the helping relationship with respect to monitoring one's own behaviour and subsequent responses to extremes of emotion. Self-monitoring ensures that one does not block patient communication and that objectivity is maintained. The difficulties identified by respondents, for example long-term exposure to emotional stress through interacting with very ill patients, may result in burn-out if not monitored carefully by an adherence to systems of clinical supervision. Some respondents' views of supervision appeared somewhat distorted and might have come from unpleasant or unhelpful personal experience. Nevertheless, clinical supervision is essential if burn-out and subjectivity are to be avoided. Good clincial supervision will offer guidance, support and understanding, and assist in maintaining effectiveness.

Collaborative working

Collaboration with other disciplines in caring has received increasing emphasis in nursing and other literature and is perceived as optimising the potential for achieving patient change and individualising packages of care. However, according to the respondents, this view could cause extreme difficulties when only the nurse was motivated to bring about sustained change. In such circumstances, outcomes are very much dependent on the nurse's competence and on patient motivation, the standard of interactions between the two and environmental factors over which no one has individual control. However, collaborative working between the patient and the nurse may in practice be difficult for a number of reasons, including the seriousness of the illness, a lack of patient insight and where the patient is compelled to receive treatment without choice by virtue of the law. Little or no headway will be made in the identification of problems without patient co-operation and sufficient evidence to inform an assessment of risk. Caution is always noted in these situations. Differing therapeutic styles were evidenced from the data and are not viewed negatively providing that interpersonal competences are effective. However, whilst all FCMHNs made reference to the success of their interventions by subjectively claiming that 'it works', it is difficult to affirm such a view without a formal validation of performance.

The FCMHN as advocate

FCMHNs demonstrated a wish to advocate on behalf of their patients, but this proved difficult in practice. The roles of forensic nurses are complicated by the power they possess with respect to patient liberty and the duty that they must exercise with regard to patient and public safety; there is always a potential to compromise the nurse–patient relationship when attempting to strike this balance. Because of the dilemmas of therapy and custody, it is questionable whether FCMHNs can truly and wholeheartedly represent the patient's views, and they may thus be better positioned to assist patient contact with able advocates.

Issues not addressed by the nurses' assessment approaches

Aspects of physical health and spiritual health were not identified in the assessment processes articulated by the nurses, leaving gaps in assessments generated. Whether these areas did not feature in the assessment process at all, or were addressed in later visits, was not established. One might be safe in assuming that patients recently discharged from hospital have received physical health checks prior to discharge, but the same may not apply to patients coming directly to the FCMHN's caseload from the community or prison. With a high prevalence of general health care problems being found in the chronically mentally ill, there is reason enough to focus on physical as well as psychological needs. CPNs and FCMHNs are in a unique position to take a lead in integrating physical health care into the assessment process in order to assist in determining the risk to physical health by screening at the earliest opportunity possible. At the very least, physical ill-health that contributes to mental disorder must be identified and appropriate treatment be arranged.

Spirituality is a poorly understood concept and is largely overlooked within the nursing literature, which may explain its lack of inclusion in the assessment process. It is nevertheless an area of need that requires exploration as it is important to many individuals and is necessary in order to achieve a holistic approach to care.

Some education and training implications

The study did not specifically elicit responses about education and training. However, many of the areas of role ambiguity, dilemma, unresolved personal conflict or practitioner need could be addressed in programmes of systematic preparation. Also, induction programmes are useful in stipulating parameters of practice, indicating sources of guidance, and in the avoidance of some elements of trial and error. Other professions and agencies may also experience confusion in relation to the role of the FCMHN, and multiagency workshops and training are essential to creating trusting and mutually respectful and informed working relationships (Campbell and Lindow, 1997).

Conclusions

The study described some of the FCMHNs' practices during their first interviews with patients. A positive message came across from all the respondents about their overall enthusiasm and motivation for their work with mentally disordered offenders. The outcome suggests that, although FCMHNs lacked guidelines and direction, they were nevertheless offering a service of some value, albeit in a rather haphazard manner. It is clear that services should offer guidance by setting parameters of approach within which desired outcomes and standards can be set, audited and further refined.

The data showed evidence of individuals working independently of each other. Approaches to assessment appeared to be self-directed, and therapeutic input was dictated by self-interest. The lack of a formal approach to assessment must bring into question the reliability of the total care package and the quality of care given, suggesting an urgent need for a standardised approach to comprehensive assessment in order to identify and manage the attendant risks in the community.

Some patients were regularly visited with the prime objective only of socialisation, the overall intent being to pursue normalisation with the individual. Admirable though this might be, it is not a viable and cost-effective way to work in the present economic climate and suggests a need for an alternative strategy. In addition to economic factors and where the ultimate aim is for socialisation to occur outside the patient's home, the practice of the FCMHN making home visits may actually impede the patient's progress.

The need for nurses to have opportunities to receive advice, support and assistance was a theme emerging from the study sample. A shared understanding of the value, utility and limitations of clinical supervision is necessary within caring organisations. This common understanding should include a shared obligation to ensure that all nurses are given the opportunity to ventilate their feelings, express their issues and concerns, share problems and develop strategies of coping. Clinical supervision may contribute towards a reduction in nurses' stress levels, ensuring that their ability to assess and treat remains effective and objective. In addition, nurses should be encouraged to develop the ability to reflect on practice and proactively embrace change and growth. This should assist in maintaining a freshness of appreciation and positive outlook.

Critical thinking skills and sound theoretical and knowledge bases are essential for competent practice. However, many nursing actions are steeped in tradition, and it would be difficult for some to justify decisions and actions as implied by the concept of accountability. Trial and error practices by FCMHNs (without a knowledge of the research findings) give cause for concern. Despite this, the FCMHNs in this study regularly referred to the success of their interventions. Whether this success arises from the effectiveness of their actions, or the effects of drug therapies, is unknown. The acquisition of a comprehensive awareness of the patient's situation will occur with systematic, reliable assessment processes. FCMHNs who have adopted standardised tools and therapeutic approaches quickly come to realise that there are common core problems that lead to standard formulations and respond to known therapeutic interventions; practices rooted in this paradigm are likely to be more acceptable when exposed to scrutiny.

This study, along with other extant evidence, suggests an urgent requirement for FCMHNs and forensic nurses generally to provide evidence of their efficiency and effectiveness. The gateway to such practice is the use of rigorous assessment materials that inform treatment formulations and predict outcomes against which measurements may be taken. Capturing the knowledge of experienced practitioners by systematic study and research will lead to a better understanding of 'how we know' when specific interventions will work. Such endeavours will only serve to identify which approaches are most effective and will ensure that FCMHNs further facilitate the exploration of the nurse–patient relationship as a therapeutic tool in itself.

References

Benner P (1984) From Novice to Expert. Wokingham: Addison Wesley.

Boyd WD (1996) Report of the Confidential Inquiry into Homicides and Suicides by Mentally Ill People. London: Royal College of Psychiatrists.

Campbell P, Lindow V (1997) Changing Practice: Mental Health Nursing and User Empowerment. London: MIND and Royal College of Nursing.

Chinn P, Jacobs M (1991) Theory and Nursing, 3rd Edn. New York: Mosby Year Book.

Cocozza JJ, Steadman HJ (1974) Some refinements in the measurement and prediction of dangerous behaviour. American Journal of Psychiatry 131(9): 1012–14.

Crichton J (1995) Psychiatric Patient Violence: Risk and Response. London: Duckworth.

Davies W, Burgess PW (1988) Prison officers' experience as a predictor of risk of attack: an analysis within the British prison system. Medicine, Science and the Law 28: 135–8.

Department of Health (1994) Working in Partnership: The Report of the Mental Health Nursing Review Team. London: HMSO.

Department of Health (1997) Developing Partnerships in Mental Health. London: HMSO.

Heron J (1975) Six Category Intervention Analysis. Guildford: Human Potential Research Project, University of Surrey.

Horder J (1992) Supervision and Counselling. London: Rochester Foundation.

Howells K, Hollin CR (Eds) (1989) Clinical Approaches to Violence. Chichester: John Wiley & Sons.

Loucas K (1982) Assessing dangerousness in psychotics. In Hamilton J, Freeman H (Eds) Dangerousness: Psychiatric Assessment and Management. London: Gaskell.

Monahan J (1981) Predicting Violent Behaviour. London: Sage.

Monahan J (1988) Risk assessment of violence among the mentally disordered: generating useful knowledge. International Journal of Law and Psychiatry 11: 249–57.

Pollock N, McBain I, Webster CD (1989) Clinical decision making and the assessment of dangerousness. In Howells K, Hollin CR (Eds) Clinical Approaches to Violence. Chichester: John Wiley & Sons.

Prins H (1990) Dangerousness – a review. In Bluglass R, Bowden R (Eds) Principles and Practice of Forensic Psychiatry. London: Churchill Livingstone.

Robinson K, Vaughan B (1992) Knowledge for Nursing Practice. London: Butterworth-Heinemann.

Rogers CR (1957) The necessary and sufficient conditions of therapeutic personality change. Journal of Consulting Psychology 21: 95–104.

Rooney J, Tarbuck P (1997) Buying Forensic Mental Health Nursing: An RCN Guide for Purchasers. London: RCN.

Scott P (1977) Assessing dangerousness in criminals. British Journal of Psychiatry 131: 127–42.

Steadman H, Cocozza J, Mellick M (1978) Explaining the increased arrest rate among mental patients: the changing clientele of state hospitals. American Journal of Psychiatry 135: 816–20.

UKCC (United Kingdom Central Council for Nursing, Midwifery and Health Visiting) (1993) Code of Professional Conduct, 3rd Edn. London: UKCC.

Chapter 6
Is high-security care necessary for persons with learning disabilities?

COLIN BEACOCK

June 25th, 1991, was a significant day for all those inhabitants of the UK who had previously been deemed mentally handicapped. It was on this day that Stephen Dorrell MP, then Secretary of State for Health, announced that henceforth such people would be described as having learning disabilities.

In the press release that announced Mr Dorrell's speech to the Mencap conference (Department of Health, 1991a), he was reported as stating that:

> Concern about the continuity of support is a major worry for many parents of people with learning disabilities. It lies at the root of concern about the closure of hospitals, and the shift to what is perceived to be less permanent forms of service provision.
>
> The need, nevertheless, is to move away from a state of affairs where reliance and trust are placed primarily in facilities; in premises, buildings or institutions which are perceived as inherently trustworthy simply because they exist and are visibly permanent. We need to move away from this towards a system which can be trusted – a system which disabled individuals and their parents or carers can trust to respond flexibly and sensitively to needs and preferences, which themselves may change significantly over time.

One major exception to this new terminology, with its more positive and humane connotations, involved those people with a mental handicap who were subjected to Sections of the Mental Health Act 1983.

Mentally disordered offenders

At law, persons with learning disability would continue to be referred to as mentally impaired or severely mentally impaired, the nomenclature adopted by the Mental Health Act 1983. These terms reinforce medical (rather than social and educational) perceptions of the developmental needs of the persons concerned. A minority of this group of the mentally impaired will have offended against the law. Therefore, some persons with a learning disability are mentally disordered offenders (MDOs), a small proportion of whom will require hospital services under conditions of security. Such facilities and services are still mainly based around the high-security hospitals at Ashworth, Broadmoor and Rampton.

The systems and facilities of the high-security hospitals are a long way removed from those described by Stephen Dorrell as evidence of enlightened practice characterised by the title 'learning disabled'. Deprived of their liberty, this client group appears to be subjected to a further social disadvantage by dint of the fact that they are classified more by their criminal or dangerous propensities than by their specific developmental needs. To entrust their care and development to services that epitomise many of the deficiencies identified by Mr Dorrell appears to be illogical, if not immoral.

The Reed Review

The Reed Review, chaired by Dr John Reed (Department of Health and Home Office, 1992), decided to establish a working group of officials who would look closely at services for MDOs with special needs, and proposed that this would include a specific review of people with learning disabilities and autism. Perhaps the most relevant recommendation of that working group was that:

> Definitive central guidance should be issued on the provision of services for offenders with learning disabilities and others requiring similar services. This should be brought to the attention of all relevant services, including criminal justice, education and housing agencies. It should take account of recommendations emerging from this review and the parallel group looking at services for people with learning disabilities and severe psychiatric or behavioural disturbance, as well as requirements set out in earlier guidance.

The very fact that it is seven years since those words were written, and that there have been no significant developments in respect of them, illustrates the urgency with which they were viewed. No central guidance has been received, nor is it imminent. What few developments have occurred have been as a result of local initiatives, using the contents of the Reed Review as basic guidance.

In considering a positive way forward, the Review identified the guiding principles as being:

- community- rather than institutionally based settings;
- conditions of security that were no greater than befitted the requirements of the individual;
- the maximising of rehabilitative opportunities with a view to fulfilling individual potential for independent living;
- a service that was as near as possible to the person's family and community.

At the same time, there was a need to expand community-based services (especially in day care), medium secure and outreach services, the academic base and research and development approaches to providing services for MDOs. The overall aim should be to reduce custodial disposal of the MDO and develop joint working between all the agencies involved.

If the rhetoric of the Reed Review appears to echo the sentiments of Stephen Dorrell's address to Mencap, this is hardly surprising. The central themes of the government's policy for health and social care are contained in the NHS and Community Care Act 1990, following on the reviews and working papers of *Working for Patients* (Department of Health, 1989) and *Caring for People* (Department of Health, 1991b). The aim is to promote a flexible health and social care service that matches resources to individual patient needs.

Assessment and management of risk

Crucial to this flexible approach is the assessment of need and the management of resources. The assessment of need for MDOs is closely linked to the assessment of risk. Where individual patients are felt to pose a risk to themselves or others, this should be reflected in the person's programme of care and rehabilitation. Systems and methods of care for such individuals must be sufficiently flexible to accommodate a wide range of needs and to allow for the risk posed by the individual to be managed in a suitable manner. The emphasis placed upon community-based care and the apparent inability of institutional care systems to provide flexible care programmes would suggest that there is little point in pursuing an argument for the relative value of hospitalised care for mentally impaired offenders.

The consideration of levels of security appropriate to the needs of the individual also begs the question of why the all-embracing security systems of high-security hospitals are felt to be suitable for the care of those with learning disabilities. The indication for placement within a high secure environment must be that the therapies and treatments pertaining to that person's behaviour (as correlated to the index offence) are only available within the high-security hospital. This would appear to be a highly questionable state of affairs given that many of those patients currently detained in high secure hospitals, and who are identified as having learning disabilities, have no index offence behaviours and are there as a legacy of previous systems of care. The likelihood of the hospitals addressing their index offences is perhaps less certain than if such people were cared for in less secure settings. In my experience, patients in high secure hospitals appear, in many cases, to be there simply because there were no appropriate alternative facilities available at the time of disposal by the courts, and there appears to be no rational explanation for why they continue to be cared for in such secure settings.

As previously mentioned, the assessment of need and the management of perceived risk are crucial in deciding the systems and settings required by the person with a learning disability. These issues are not exclusive to people who are described as mentally impaired offenders but to all people with a learning disability. As the traditional hospital-based services have declined, and a more socially appropriate system of care has been developed in community settings, care teams have been called upon to make complex decisions with, and on behalf of, service users. There is an immediate and inherent risk in removing any individual from a closed institutional setting to one which brings them more closely into the focus of mainstream society. The programme of integration and preparation depends upon a two-way learning process involving the individual client and the community, one encompassing joint approaches to the management of risk. For example, although the Reed Review indicates the desirability of having services in close proximity to the person's family, it may not be desirable that a person with a learning disability (who is a mentally impaired offender) who significantly offended the community should receive care within that community as the risk posed to the programme of rehabilitation may be significant in such circumstances. So, if the principles of the Reed Review cannot be enacted, where are such 'outcasts' to go?

From the comments made by Stephen Dorrell, it would appear that the concept of specialised communities, such as those established by Home Farm Trust, Mencap and other voluntary and charitable groups, have no specific role to play unless their services are relevant to the developmental needs of the individual. Co-operation between agencies and authorities is an increasing feature of service provision and is encouraged within the Reed Review. Partnerships between health and social care providers in the private, voluntary and statutory sectors are increasing phenomena emerging from the development of services based around the NHS and Community Care Act. It may well be that services for people with learning disabilities (who are mentally impaired offenders) will reflect that trend.

Code of practice

In the Mental Health Act Code of Practice (Department of Health and Welsh Office, 1993), there is a section devoted specifically to the needs of persons with a learning disability. Here, the relevance of assessment of need is emphasised, and the Code of Practice advises that:

> The assessment of a person with learning disabilities requires special considera-
> tion to be given to communication with the person being assessed. Wherever
> possible the ASW (Approved Social Worker) should have had experience of
> working with people with learning disabilities or be able to call upon someone
> who has.

The glib nature of this statement is a cause for major concern. How can a social worker be approved to assess a person when he or she may have had *experience* but no specialist training or education in the care and management of the client group being assessed? The very idea is scandalous, especially given that the outcome of the assessment may well result in a loss of liberty for the person being assessed. The Code of Practice appears to recognise that holders of the Certificate of Qualification in Social Work need not have had any substantial experience with this client group, except that gained in pre-certification training. Holders of the more recently introduced Diploma in Social Work would only have greater insight if this client group fell into one of their areas of special interest. What better case can there be for a revision of the Mental Health Act 1983 to recognise the registered nurse for the mentally handicapped as an 'approved social worker' within the context of the Act?

Challenging behaviours

Where a person with a learning disability displays violent, aggressive or antisocial behaviour, he or she is said to challenge the resources of society. Such people are deemed to have a *health* rather than a *social care* need. This concept leaves much to be desired since many of the behaviours that individuals and groups have developed occur in direct response to their having been subjected to those institutional practices which masqueraded as health care regimes. Nonetheless, in 1990, the Chief Nursing Officers of the UK commissioned a report to examine the future role of the registered nurse for the mentally handicapped within the context of *Caring for People* (Department of Health, 1991b). Chaired by Professor Chris Cullen, the report stated that:

> Health professionals are needed to ensure that health, in the World Health Organisation sense of 'a state of complete physical, mental and social well-being' is maintained as a top priority for people with mental handicaps ... there are undoubtedly many clients who will only need opportunities for ordinary living and access to ordinary facilities to achieve this state. However, there are many, especially those who have significant physical disabilities, sensory problems or challenging behaviour, who will sometimes require the services of skilled professionals in order to help them to benefit from non-institutionalised living. This is where we see the role of nurses and other health professionals.

Such a definition of role would appear to have relevance to the development of services envisaged by both Reed and Dorrell. Where individuals have displayed offence behaviours, they may be seen as displaying challenging behaviours but have no clearly defined health care needs. It is in such circumstances that a re-evaluation of what constitutes health and/or social need is required. Court diversion schemes may well prevent custodial sentences, but these offenders (or defendants) undoubtedly require a programme of social education, therapy and (occasionally) medical treatment that will enable their rehabilitation into society.

Previous concepts of health care and treatment need to be re-examined in light of the World Health Organisation definition and new ideas adopted so that only the very few patients whose patterns of behaviour might indicate a requirement for high-security services are referred there. In such circumstances, the period of high secure stay should be for no longer than was indicated by individual need. For those people who are currently in receipt of high-security services because of the threat they pose to themselves and others (even though they have committed no index offence), their needs for such an individualised programme are equally justified. Indeed, where such people have made little or no progress over a number of years, there is a self-evident case for saying that they are inappropriately placed. Where these people have been on waiting lists for discharge over a number of years, they are being neglected by society, and their basic human rights are being seriously infringed.

Service developments

In order to make best use of the learning potential offered by community-based programmes, carers would need to have a skills base that reflected high levels of transferability based upon interpersonal and re-educative principles. The developmental delays of the client would indicate that they might well require a life-long programme of learning for health. It may be argued that such an approach is more easily provided within the confines of an institutional setting and that economies of scale are essential within financial reality. Such decisions must be made solely on the grounds of individual needs and risk assessment. Services for this client group have always and will continue to represent a high-cost investment. What is required is a realignment so that the resources of the Exchequer are invested in developing a flexible service with carers, rather than facilities, as its core resource.

It is the concept of 'investment' that must underpin the development of a future service for this client group. Existing returns on investment, if viewed in terms of recovery rate (with regard to non-recidivism) and duration of rehabilitation (in terms of discharge to areas of lower security), do not appear to be very high. The wasted investment tied down in providing inappropriately high levels of security indicates that there is an opportunity cost factor that suggests that these resources might be better invested elsewhere. Shiell and Wright (1988) examined the costs of community care and concluded that:

> the larger residential setting is obviously not as expensive as its smaller counter-part but this does not mean that it is necessarily more efficient. Efficiency describes the relationship between costs and effect. A cost-effective service is not necessarily one that minimises cost per se but one which minimises the cost of achieving a given level of benefit. Cost is therefore only one determinant of efficiency and it is equally important to consider the effect the use of services has on clients and their families. Thus, the quality of care and ultimately its impact on the user's quality of life must also be assessed.

The assertion that high-security services, such as are currently being provided, are a cost-effective method of provision would appear to be at odds with the views of Shiell and Wright. The backlog of people awaiting discharge alone would appear to provide sufficient evidence to support the argument that the opportunity to reinvest significant levels of resources is being prevented because society is supporting an outmoded and inappropriate system of provision.

Such security as is required by the majority of this client group is relational in nature; that is to say, it depends heavily upon the therapeutic and developmental relationship that evolves between client and carer. When standards and practice are driven by changing needs of the individual client and are monitored and assessed by a multidisciplinary care team – whose leader has a co-ordinatory rather than a clinical role – the system of health care becomes less dependent upon facilities and more dependent upon the care process. When the overall outcome of that process of health care is the integration of the client into a support system that maximises his or her level of independent functioning, there is an ultimate target against which to measure achievements.

What results would be a cycle of care that addresses changing needs in an evolutionary manner and within which decision-making is based upon evidence drawn from meaningful, focused reports. Levels of security would form but one part of the overall assessment of needs. This is in contrast to the legacy of Victorian values that constitutes our existing facilities and systems.

Conclusions

From the arguments presented, the answer to the question that opened this chapter is that high-security care *is* evidently necessary for those with learning disabilities, but only as one very small part of an integrated system of developmental care. The institutional component should be of the smallest possible unit size, and the security must be of high intensity for as short a duration as is required by the person involved. The basic assumption is that society actually wishes to rehabilitate mentally impaired offenders and those people with a learning disability who pose a significant risk to themselves and others. Then again, if it is punishment you are after, the Victorians, with their large institutions, appear to have got things about right!

References

Department of Health (1989) Working for Patients. London: HMSO.
Department of Health (1991a) Stephen Dorrell announces publication of guidance on facilities for people with Learning Disabilities. HC 91/286. London: Department of Health.
Department of Health (1991b) Caring for People: Mental Handicap Nursing. London: HMSO.

Department of Health and Home Office (1992) Review of Health and Social Services
    for Mentally Disordered Offenders and Others Requiring Similar Services
(The Reed Review). Cmnd 2088. London: HMSO.
Department of Health and Welsh Office (1993) Code of Practice: Mental Health Act
    1983. Section 118. London: HMSO.
Shiell A, Wright K (1988) Counting the Cost of Community Care. York: University of
    York.

Chapter 7
Crime, mental disorder and criminology: a critical perspective

DAVID MERCER

> Criminological theories which seemed to recognise the social basis for crime were all the rage in universities, but the models accepted and utilised by the prison service were rooted in the stigmatising concepts of forensic psychiatry. (Reeve, 1983)

The 'dilemma of therapeutic custody' for nursing staff working in the Special Hospitals is well documented in current discourse and debate (Burrow, 1991; Tarbuck, 1994). Indeed, in both structural and symbolic terms, these archetypal, 'total', institutions represent and reify the medico-legal interface. Casting a shadow across the divided camps of those who champion reform and those who advocate abolition, their walls are a stark and visible manifestation of society's response to the mentally disordered offender.

Yet, this is both a history and a legacy. The political and professional language of deinstitutionalisation, and an expansion of regional services/units, evidence a development of, rather than a break from, this tradition. If the Special Hospital nurse has metamorphosed into the forensic psychiatric practitioner, the role remains a 'corollary of the "*medicalisation of criminology*"' (Richman and Mason, 1992, emphasis added). A sophistication in the organisation and technology of treatment/intervention may deliver us from the controlled environment into the controlling community, but it also ushers in 'a new ideology of control in which society itself becomes more and more like a closed institution' (Schrag, 1980).

This chapter seeks to explore the relationship between crime and mental disorder by focusing on the criminological enterprise not as an objective body of knowledge, but as a powerful force in shaping theory, research, policy and practice.

71

The forensic factor

The fundamental contradiction and challenge of forensic nursing, then, irrespective of the specific location of that practice, is the duality of 'mental illness' and 'criminal behaviour' in a single patient/client population. In the clinical field and the classroom alike, a commonality of questions emerges centred upon the convergence of, and connections between, *disease* and *deviance*, as does a concern about the most appropriate target for nursing intervention, that is, should it be symptom and/or offence related? It is largely the criminogenic component – embracing the construct of 'dangerousness' – that has dogged the introduction of innovative generic approaches into secure settings (Mason and Chandley, 1990) and prompted the development of exclusively forensic models of care (Tarbuck, 1994).

That nursing, akin to medicine, is an activity that professes to be directed at the *individual* calls for a critical appraisal of criminological theory as part of the emerging 'scientific' knowledge base of forensic staff. The essential issue here concerns the delivery rather than the design of a curriculum. To explore the nature of crime is, assuredly, a vital role of courses such as the ENB's 'Nursing in Controlled Environments' (ENB 770) or their higher educational successors at diploma or degree level. However, the framing of the questions that are asked need to confront, rather than complement, the traditional philosophy of nurse training, a dichotomy ideally illustrated by the search for a relationship between criminality and mental illness.

If the origins of professional nursing derive from the works of Nightingale (Tarbuck, 1994), the ideological framework of thought and practice is firmly rooted in the medical reductionism of the nineteenth-century asylum. It is suggested that the functional value of our early ancestors was to enhance the power of physicians in contrast to establishing a distinctive nursing identity, which, at the same time, 'did not progress care of the mentally ill because their training did not imply or encourage questioning of the *positivistic* basis of psychiatric treatment' (Chung and Nolan, 1994, emphasis added). Shifting attention from the language of causation to that of context, or from cure to control, is to begin unravelling the interwoven ideologies that underpin mental health and criminal justice, and, in so doing, move us towards a 'history of the present' (Foucault, 1977).

As Blackburn (1993) notes, 'the relationship between mental disorder and crime reflects changing interactions between criminal justice and mental health systems as much as *scientific* concern' (emphasis added). Yet, the quest to identify an aetiological link between two distinct human experiences or variables (mental illness and criminality) has overshadowed the larger issue of social construction mediated by professional power (Ingleby, 1985). However, a number of seminal works, rekindling and revitalising the libertarian critique of the 1960s, have laid the foundations for a critical analysis of the medical appropriation of insanity and crime. Iconoclastic histories of the asylum and the penitentiary (Foucault, 1973, 1977; Ignatieff, 1978) counter the received wisdom of compassion, reform and neutrality whilst illuminating the operation of state institutions in contemporary society. Although the theoretical perspectives of the authors differ, these writers 'emphasised a historical position that eschewed benevolent progression for more structural dimensions of political economy, social class, ideology and power' (Sim, 1990). The genesis of psychiatry and medicine in the prisons and mad-houses of the eighteenth century was inextricably linked to the maintenance of order amidst a new set of capitalist social relations.

Medicine and madness

Explanations of disease and illness have varied over time and between cultures. Until the late eighteenth century, European medicine comprised a combination of both 'personalistic' and 'naturalistic' systems, respectively seeing sickness as the result of external forces or an internal imbalance of body elements (Morgan et al, 1985). A changing conceptualisation of disease, as being aetiologically specific and universal, accompanied the consolidation of professional medicine based upon the scientific paradigm; from the early nineteenth century, the biomedical model assumed a dominance that has continued into the present. Diagnostic taxonomies and curative interventions 'resulted in health and illness being seen in *individualistic* terms, with the causes of illness and responsibility for health largely residing with the individual' (Morgan et al, 1985, emphasis added). Although it is generally portrayed as the triumph of rational knowledge, critics have pointed to the social factors and forces that shaped the ascendancy of medical power; that disease categories, rather than existing 'out there' to be discovered and defined, independently of the physician/doctor, are socially interpreted and constructed (Freidson, 1970; Illich, 1975).

In terms of 'mental illness', orthodox texts likewise suggest that the 'nineteenth-century take-over of the field by medicine, and its consolidation in recent years, demonstrate the progressive spread in our society of principles of reason and humanity' (Ingleby, 1985). Critical histories, in stark contrast however, have vigorously attacked the application of medical metaphor and methods to 'diseases of the mind', articulated vociferously in the anti-psychiatry school (Goffman, 1961; Laing and Esterson, 1964) and claimed for a 'therapeutic state' (Kittrie, 1971). Indeed, for Conrad and Schneider (1980), the historical development of 'mental illness' is 'literally the original case of *medicalised deviance*' (emphasis added).

The emergence of a unitary concept of mental illness, and the expanded psychiatric nosology of Kraeplin and Bleuler, derived from the philosophical tenets of positivism – the idea that the social world, like the natural world, was accessible to empirical investigation, measurement, prediction and control. These intellectual pioneers exerted an immense influence over the administration and organisation of the asylums and the work that went on within them, particularly that of nurses, status and control being embodied in a rigid division of labour between those who observed (collected) data and those who owned (analysed) it. The servility of asylum attendants became the subservience of nursing: 'Nurses' induction into the positivistic tradition was allowed to take them only as far as would maintain the hierarchy of the asylum system' (Chung and Nolan, 1994).

Despite these advances in diagnostic classification, they were unsupported by either somatic pathology or effective treatment. Ironically, medical prestige was enhanced by an investment of faith in the scientific method rather than any demonstration of its validity; the objectivity and value freedom of physicians remained unchallenged as madness was defined in medical language. Graphic examples such as 'drapetomania' (Fernando, 1992) – an 'illness' that caused slaves to run away from plantations – illustrate well, however, the Eurocentric, imperialist infrastructure of the nascent discipline; exploitation and oppression were alien concepts to the alienists. 'Disease' labels could be attached to any behaviour at variance with a particular and normative view of the world, including crime (Conrad and Schneider, 1980). For Szasz (1961; 1970), 'mental illness' becomes a manufactured 'myth', with a powerful ideological impact upon the management and control of human difference. The quest for organic explanations is, in this sense, an illusory exercise. For even if such a causal connection were established, it could not 'alter the fact that it was social, political or cultural criteria which defined the deviance in the first place' (Schrag, 1980).

This debate clearly assumes a key prominence as we move towards a consideration of the role of medicine in relation to *legal* or *moral* transgression. One aspect of the 'sick role' (Parsons, 1951) is to excuse the individual, dependent upon their acceptance of the illness label and appropriate treatment, from responsibility or blame. For Szasz (1961), the enforcement of this complicated equation is a fundamental assault on freedom, dignity and human rights. Others, in contrast, have postulated that those deemed 'insane' should be exempted from culpability and punishment, based upon a want of reason, and not because of any analogy between physical disease and madness. This philosophical position is central to the classic legal definition of the McNaghten Rules, and ongoing controversy about the attribution of (diminished) responsibility, particularly in relation to 'psychopathic' offenders (Bavidge, 1989). The methodological problems, and exclusivity, of research that attempts to identify 'isolable variables' in order to explain functional or psychotic 'conditions' have been noted (Coulter, 1973; Sheldon, 1984). Coulter notes that 'it is precisely where *beliefs* are taken as "symptoms" of some undiscovered biological abnormality that the solitary individual organism model peculiar to biogenetic work encounters most trouble' (Coulter, 1973, emphasis added). Profound differences, however, are obscured by an association between 'mental illness' and 'medical science', which is both an 'idea' and an 'ideology', insulating psychiatry from the focus of critical inquiry (Leifer, 1969).

Suggestions that the development of psychotherapeutic approaches represents an emancipatory break from the past similarly warrant closer scrutiny. It has been argued that the contribution of Freud merely shifted the 'dialogue' from 'biogenic determinism' to 'psychogenic determinism' (Conrad and Schneider, 1980), extending the medical model of madness to a wider range of deviant behaviour and emotional problems. The historical and cultural construction of hysteria, which remains contested as a disease category, is illustrative of connections between clinical practice, sexual division and patriarchal culture, introducing into the analysis the structural dimension of gender (Showalter, 1987). If women who dare to affront the norms and role expectations of a male-dominated society are less obviously suppressed by contemporary psychiatry, medical knowledge reflects and reinforces popular prejudice. Also, it is another irony that the profession that for so long actively silenced the voices of female survivors of sexual abuse (Masson, 1985, 1990; Salter, 1990) should transform into their therapeutic salvation.

The discourse that emphasises personal pathology in abused and battered women, according them the status of 'patient' or 'client', has been accompanied by a massive escalation in the numbers of those allied to the mental health movement – clinical psychologists, family therapists and an army of counsellors (Dobash and Dobash, 1992).

Political and economic problems are masked by clinical language, and change equates with the process of individual therapy. Paralleling the institutional confinement of the nineteenth century, it is, again, a change of 'tactic' rather than 'strategy' (Ingleby, 1985). This is both the promise and the problem of the 'therapeutic society': 'The objective now appears to be perfection of self through psychotherapy and counselling' (Dobash and Dobash, 1992). To discuss the lives of the marginalised – the mentally ill and the criminal – without questioning our own lives is sadly short-sighted.

Medicine and crime

In the discussion so far, attention has been directed towards the blurring of boundaries, and degree of merger, between the 'criminal justice' and 'mental health' systems, generating in the 1960s and 70s a growing concern about the 'medicalisation of deviance' as a mode of social control. Examples have already been cited from an ever-extending list of behaviours, previously understood in legal or moral terms, which have transferred into the medical arena. Along with the victims of domestic violence and child abuse, we can include the perpetrators of those acts and other forms of sexual offending, drug addiction, alcoholism, prostitution and political dissent (Miller, 1980). Indeed, from shoplifting to serial killing, the expertise of the psychiatrist can be invoked and the concept of punishment replaced with that of treatment. To begin asking why this should be so is to explore the nature of both crime and criminology as the important question about relationhips between criminality and mental disorder is an ideological one and is again rooted in history.

As for madness, the definitions of deviance (the transgression of societal values) and crime (the transgression of criminal law) have varied over time and between cultures, as have the types of sanction and punishment meted out in response to socially proscribed behaviour. Explanations of infraction and offending, and particular forms of control, reflect historically specific mechanisms for managing human difference: religion (founded on faith), law (founded on a legal code) and, latterly, medicine (founded on science) (Miller,

1980). These conflicting, and at times entangled, systems of social control have important, practical ramifications for the disposal and treatment of deviant individuals, embracing larger debates about retribution, reform and rehabilitation.

Criminology has broadly been defined as 'the study of crime, of attempts to control it, and of attitudes to it' (Walker, 1983). Although this concise description adequately outlines the administrative mainstream of the discipline, it obscures external influences and internal contradictions. As Young (1988) points out, 'criminology does not occur in a vacuum'. Traditionally, then, criminological research, controlled and constrained by the state, has been dominated by twin concerns: to locate the cause of crime at an individual level, and to improve the operational effectiveness of the criminal justice agencies (Young, 1981). In idealising the major theoretical paradigms in criminological thinking, the latter author examines each model in terms of its conception of human nature, social order, ideas about causation and policy implications, concluding that the definitional variability of 'crime' makes an all-encompassing, unitary theory improbable (Young, 1981). The recognition that *all* criminology is political is a pivotal position in more recent 'radical' and 'critical' perspectives. Offering a challenge to correctional criminology – 'the face of the enemy' (Hester and Eglin, 1992) – they have attempted to construct a 'fully social theory of deviance' to 'demonstrate theoretically the connections between law and the state, legal and political relations, the economic basis and functions of crime' (Hall and Scraton, 1981).

The historical development of criminology is inextricably linked to the 'positivist revolution' initiating a tradition of research and theory, grounded in the nineteenth-century institutional structures of the asylum and the prison; Bluglass (1980) notes how the genesis of forensic psychiatry is linked to early attempts to establish a 'scientific criminology'. An understanding of these changes in the organisation of penology has to be located in the wider social relations of a society undergoing radical change. During the eighteenth century, crime, in the 'classicist' sense, was interpreted as a rational activity, deliberately chosen, based upon a calculus of odds. Correspondingly, justice – embodied in the notion of 'social contract' – sought deterrence, through a scale of penalties proportional to the degree of harm produced. Thus, the individual was seen as being responsible for his or her actions and was punished accordingly (Young, 1981).

Writing from a Marxist perspective, Melossi and Pavarini (1981) made a pioneering contribution to our understanding of the 'real' connections between prisons and the social structure. Their histori-

cal analysis is written against the backdrop of increasing ferment and
protest within a penal system in 'crisis' throughout the Western
world. Prior to the nineteenth century, little use was made of impris-
onment, the main forms of punishment – as a public spectacle –
including whipping, branding and execution (Giddens, 1994). It was
the breakdown of feudalism and the emergence of a capitalist economy that gave birth to the modern penitentiary and, more importantly, the penalty of confinement as a deprivation of liberty (Melossi
and Pavarini, 1981). Whereas the privation of socially valued assets
(money, status, life, etc.) had previously sufficed, a new form of
retributive punishment was required commensurate with exchange
value and waged labour, representing, that is, a clear relationship
between the means of production and the means of punishment.
Thus, it is argued, 'in every industrial society, the institution has
become the dominant punitive instrument to such an extent that
prison and punishment are commonly regarded as almost synony-
mous' (Melossi and Pavarini, 1981).

As criminality and madness merged with the disease epidemics
that followed industrialisation, 'confinement' became part of a
changing discourse about public hygiene based upon a surveillance
of points of contact between the individual and the societal body
(Foucault, 1973). The disciplinary regime of the penitentiary paral-
leled the 'moral therapy' of the asylum, both sharing a concern
about maintaining social order through a resocialisation of reason in
inmates and felons (Ignatieff, 1978, 1981). Often interpreted as the
symbolic turning point in enlightened care, the reforms of Pinel and
Tuke represent the triumph of medicine over crime and insanity.
These measures witnessed an expansion, and legitimation, of 'discipline' to embrace the mind as well as the body, one 'intended to
transform the mad, sad and bad into the disciplined and docile
workforce required for the purposes of industrial capitalism (Dobash
and Dobash, 1992).

It was in these carceral institutions that criminologists such as
Caesare Lombroso commenced their search for the 'criminal man'
as doctors and jurors wrestled for possession of the 'dangerous individual' (Foucault, 1978). Founded on the theoretical and pragmatic
tenets of positivism – identification, quantification, prediction and
control – this early work crystallised the idea of criminality as individual, innate and inherited. Crime had been redefined as a 'disease'
committed by those abnormal in body or mind; punishment, no
longer appropriate, was replaced with indeterminate detention for
treatment. At the same time, the focus of the analysis shifted atten-

tion away from the contextual structure in which human action took place, and away from any human meaning attached to it.

Although now obsolete relics of the past, the early ideas of 'stigmata' and 'atavism' that characterise the 'born criminal' are echoed in a lineage of the 'scientific' testing of incarcerated populations (Sapsford, 1981); nursing staff certainly do not have to rely on television drama to be introduced to the terrifying figure of the 'XYY man'. Depending upon fashion, and technology, prisoners have, as Box (1981) notes, 'had their heads measured for irregularities, their bodies somatotyped, their unconscious's probed and analysed, their intelligence rated, their personalities typed, their brains scanned, and their gene structure investigated', research that has to date yielded, at best, inconclusive and contested data. And yet, as in *Star Trek*, the quest continues ... with a growing list of 'reified pseudo-medical abstractions': violence, aggression, personality disorder, etc. (Schrag, 1980). As the barrage of tests swell in number, science defines morality and claims the soul of the deviant.

Conclusions

The foregoing text represents an attempt to identify the ideological connections between crime and mental disorder as they have been constructed by a dominant tradition in criminology – individual positivism. Those who would dismiss it as 'partisan' should need little reminding that all research and theory is political. The value of a Foucauldian analysis is not only the insight it gives into the 'truth' that flows from powerful institutions, but also the opportunity to challenge it. As nurses working with the most powerless, and marginalised, members of our society, this reminds us that there are other voices. The type of criminology advocated here is not an equivalent of the DSM-IV (American Psychiatric Association, 1994) – a 'do-it-yourself' kit for care-planning. Instead, it urges us to look critically at the institutions in which we work, the technology of control we use, the labels we apply and the value system that underpins all of these. There is optimism in Sim's (1990) observation that 'opposition cannot be reduced to the notion of class struggle but includes women struggling against male power, the mentally ill against psychiatric power and sections of the population against medical power'. Speaking and writing is part of that struggle.

References

American Psychiatric Association (1994) Diagnostic and Statistical Manual of Mental Disorders (DSM-IV). Washington, DC: APA.

Bavidge M (1989) Mad or Bad? Bristol: Bristol Classical Press.

Blackburn R (1993) The Psychology of Criminal Conduct: Theory, Practice and Research. Chichester: John Wiley & Sons.

Bluglass R (1980) Psychiatry, the Law and the Offender – Present Dilemmas and Future Prospects. London: Institute for the Study and Treatment of Delinquency.

Box S (1981) Deviance, Reality and Society, 2nd Edn. London: Holt, Rinehart & Winston.

Burrow S (1991) The Special Hospital nurse and the dilemma of therapeutic custody. Journal of Advances in Health and Nursing Care 1(3): 21–38.

Chung M, Nolan P (1994) The influence of positivistic thought on nineteenth century asylum nursing. Journal of Advanced Nursing 19(2): 226–32.

Conrad P, Schneider J (1980) Deviance and Medicalisation: From Badness to Sickness. London: CV Mosby.

Coulter J (1973) Approaches to Insanity. Oxford: Martin Robertson.

Dobash R, Dobash R (1992) Women, Violence and Social Change. London: Routledge.

Fernando S (1992) Roots of racism. Open Mind 59: 10–11.

Foucault M (1973) The Birth of the Clinic: An Archaeology of Medical Perception. London: Tavistock.

Foucault M (1977) Discipline and Punish: The Birth of the Prison. London: Penguin.

Foucault M (1978) About the concept of the 'dangerous individual' in 19th century legal psychiatry. International Journal of Law and Psychiatry 1: 1–18.

Freidson E (1970) Professional Dominance. New York: Atherton.

Giddens A (1994) Sociology, 2nd Edn. London: Polity Press.

Goffman E (1961) Asylums: Essays on the Social Control of Mental Patients and Other Inmates. Harmondsworth: Penguin.

Hall S, Scraton P (1981) Law, class and control. In Fitzgerald M, McLennan G, Pawson J (Eds) Crime and Society: Readings in History and Theory. London: Routledge & Kegan Paul.

Hester S, Eglin P (1992) A Sociology of Crime. London: Routledge.

Ignatieff M (1978) A Just Measure of Pain: The Penitentiary in the Industrial Revolution 1750–1850. New York: Columbia University Press.

Ignatieff M (1981) The ideological origins of the penitentiary. In Fitzgerald M, McLennan G, Pawson J (Eds) Crime and Society: Readings in History and Theory. London: Routledge & Kegan Paul.

Illich I (1975) Limits to Medicine. London: Marion Boyars.

Ingleby D (1985) Mental health and social order. In Cohen S, Scull A (Eds) Social Control and the State. Oxford: Basil Blackwell.

Kittrie N (1971) The Right to be Different: Deviance and Enforced Therapy. London: John Hopkins Press.

Laing R, Esterson R (1964) Sanity, Madness and the Family: Families of Schizophrenics. Harmondsworth: Penguin.

Leifer R (1969) The Medical Model as Idea and Ideology. New York: Science House.

Mason T, Chandley M (1990) Nursing models in a Special Hospital: a critical analysis of efficacity. Journal of Advanced Nursing 15(6): 667–73.

Masson J (1985) The Assault on Truth: Freud's Suppression of the Seduction Theory. Harmondsworth: Penguin Books.

Masson J (1990) Against Therapy. London: Fontana.

Melossi D, Pavarini M (1981) The Prison and the Factory: Origins of the Penitentiary System. London: Macmillan.

Miller K (1980) Criminal Justice and Mental Health. London: Free Press.

Morgan M, Calnan M, Manning N (1985) Sociological Approaches to Health and Medicine. London: Croom Helm.

Parsons T (1951) The social system. London: Routledge & Kegan Paul.

Reeve A (1983) Notes from a Waiting Room: Anatomy of a Political Prisoner. London: Heretic Books.

Richman J, Mason T (1992) Quo vadis the Special Hospitals? In Scott S, Williams G, Platt S, Thomas H (Eds) Private Risks and Public Dangers. Aldershot: Averbury.

Salter A (1990) Foreword. In O'Connell A, Leberg E, Donaldson C (Eds) Working with Sex Offenders: Guidelines for Therapist Selection. London: Sage.

Sapsford R (1981) Individual deviance: the search for the criminal personality. In Fitzgerald M, McLennan G, Pawson J (Eds) Crime and Society: Readings in History and Theory. London: Routledge & Kegan Paul.

Schrag P (1980) Mind Control. London: Marion Boyars.

Sheldon B (1984) A critical appraisal of the medical model in psychiatry. In Olsen M (Ed.) Social Work and Mental Health. London: Tavistock.

Showalter E (1987) The Female Malady: Women, Madness and English Culture 1830–1980. London: Virago.

Sim J (1990) Medical Power in Prisons: The Prison Medical Service in England 1774–1989. Milton Keynes: Open University Press.

Szasz T (1961) The Myth of Mental Illness: Foundations of a Theory of Personal Conduct. New York: Hoeber–Harper.

Szasz T (1970) The Manufacture of Madness: A Comparative Study of the Inquisition and the Mental Health Movement. New York: Harper & Row.

Tarbuck P (1994) The therapeutic use of security: a model for forensic nursing. In Thompson T, Mathias P (Eds) Lyttle's Mental Health and Disorder, 2nd Edn. London: Baillière Tindall.

Walker N (1983) Criminology. In Walsh D, Poole A (Eds) A Dictionary of Criminology. London: Routledge & Kegan Paul.

Young J (1981) Thinking seriously about crime: some models of criminology. In Fitzgerald M, McLennan G, Pawson J (Eds) Crime and Society: Readings in History and Theory. London: Routledge & Kegan Paul.

Young J (1988) Radical criminology in Britain: the emergence of a competing paradigm. British Journal of Criminology 28(2): 159–83.

Chapter 8
The sharp end of Broadmoor: a look at developments in nursing at Broadmoor Hospital from a patient's perspective

'HARRY'

The following chapter is adapted from an address I made at a forensic nurses' conference in November 1994. It is my experience of being a patient in Broadmoor hospital from 1988 to 1994.

As a man, I have not been able to reflect as much as I would like on some of the changes going on in the other side of the hospital – 'the female wing', as it is still known. Having said that, the changes on the male side over the past few years have reached all parts of the hospital to differing degrees. A service user's voice is imperative to measure the service provided, and this chapter is but a small part of that.

Service user involvement

There has been, as far as I can tell, a great new movement of service ex-users (and indeed users of psychiatric services) to become involved in care, treatment, advocacy and other related matters. For myself, I must emphasise that I speak as a user of forensic services with all that I carry with me. I will, however, do my best to remain objective. I do not represent patients from Broadmoor: I speak on my own behalf. Having said that, I have, in writing this chapter, drawn on the experience of fellow patients and also nurses.

In my 6 years at Broadmoor, I saw many changes in the staff culture that have gone a long way to make the place more friendly and easier to live in. My own experience has been formed from three wards and as a member of the only Patients' Equal Opportunities Committee within the Special Hospital system. Many matters came to my attention in this role. For 3 years, I was an editor of the patients' magazine, which involved interviewing people such as Home Office civil servants, John Bowis MP (the then junior Health Minister), Lord Longford, members of the Special Hospitals Service Authority and local management. A great deal has also been learnt from being a member of a unique writing venture with nurses, run by a professor in English. The papers we discussed ranged from grief counselling and professional responses to self-harm, to quality assurance.

I have no experience of any other forensic services, other than a prison hospital wing, so you will have to forgive me if my approach is focused on Broadmoor. Added to this are insights gained from experiences I had when working in care settings prior to my breakdown and subsequent admission to Broadmoor.

I have found, from listening to comments, that nurses often feel threatened by users' organisations such as MIND. It is my experience that there is room for massive improvement as the old nursing ethics and regimes are nudged aside. It was not all bad in the past though – and I ask you to consider how nurses currently practising will be judged in 30 years time. Will we have gone forward, or into more difficulties and restrictions caused by a lack of government funding? There is, of course, also widespread public ignorance of mental health issues, fuelled by the media's distorted reporting, to think about.

Patients' Council

The present Patients' Council user representative body in Broadmoor is at a very early stage of development. Making plenty of noise and being challenging in a positive way. I ask that you forget the noise and concentrate on what is being said. Much of our experience needs to be heard and discussed to enable the movement to grow – practitioners have to learn about their own methods and the way in which they interact with patients. There has for a long time been in Broadmoor, although I cannot speak for other establishments, a core of what I can only see as negative nurses, who see the emergence of patients from oppression as very threatening to their place in the establishment. They can no longer act out their high judgements. In light of this, it is enlightened nurses who must influence the direction

of forensic nursing into the next century. Massive demands will
continue to be made. Change will be necessary, and hopefully most
of it will be positive.

Changes at Broadmoor Hospital

The changes in Broadmoor since 1988 have been profound, those
which, in my opinion, have had the most impact occurring in the
following areas:

- the use of seclusion;
- 24 hour care;
- the integration of wards;
- primary nursing;
- partnerships in care;
- the nursing ethos;
- drama;
- the Snoezelen Rompa room;
- the complaints procedure.

Use of seclusion

Probably the most powerful subject to begin with is the alteration in
the use of seclusion. The changes have occurred in a place where
patients have died in seclusion rooms in controversial circumstances.
Seclusion was more often used as a punitive measure and had very
far-reaching consequences, for both patients and nurses. A punishment. For a woman to be stripped naked while male nurses were
present and left for days without contact with friends was often the
norm. No cigarettes, filthy smelly rooms, humiliation and degrada-
tion – total. It was common for a patient to be secluded for just
swearing at a charge nurse. A disturbing picture. With this in mind, it
is easy to see how the disappearance of this practice has helped to
reduce a climate of fear and oppression. I believe that personal
growth occurs much more readily in favourable conditions, and this
change has to be one of the greatest. In comparison, seclusion is
seldom used these days, and I know that some would like to see it
phased out completely. However, when one considers how damaging
a person can be, and how disruptive on a ward, it is worth considering whether it is necessary on some wards, in limited circumstances.
    On the other hand, seclusion can be very valuable. I can recall

being locked up in seclusion because of industrial action and thoroughly enjoying the experience. A bit of solitude, a bit of peace and quiet away from the noisy, crowded ward was a luxurious event. For someone who is at their wits' end, going into seclusion can be invaluable, often being taken away from the immediate cause of their distress and given time to 'get their head together'. I remember certain disturbed individuals being encouraged to go for a 'lie down' and everyone being better for it, not least that person; quite often, the door was not even locked.

The change in the use of seclusion can lead to more trust being invested in nurses (if they also are prepared to change – and in Broadmoor many have). If one can express anger and frustration without being surrounded by nurses summoned as a result of the fear engendered by raised voices, a healthier relationship of communication can be encouraged: a more appropriate way of handling a distressed or simply angry person – as was borne out for me by a much more relaxed atmosphere about the hospital – more give and take.

Along with the drop in the use of seclusion, there is the change of allowing one to speak one's mind with much less fear, and this change in the culture brings the benefit of allowing people to be themselves.

Twenty-four hour care

The practice of, for much of the hospital, locking people away in rooms or dormitories from 9 p.m. until 7 a.m. is being phased out. This is of great benefit, allowing more choice, self-responsibility and opportunity for socialising, support and getting away, as much as we can, from the negative nature of incarceration. There is, however, a downside to this new freedom of choice, for example some patients who stay up all night making a noise and being in no fit state to do anything during the day. There needs to be a constant addressing of this problem on an individual basis rather than blanket rules being imposed. On some wards, such as the intensive care wards at Broadmoor, I think it is prudent to think carefully about how this practice is used, as 24 hour care could mean 24 hour disturbance.

Integration of wards

During my time in Broadmoor, there were no integrated wards, apart from the infirmary – in practice that worked successfully. The main move now is for female nurses to enter male wards, something historically frowned upon. The opposite is also happening to a lesser degree on the female side, although men have for many years routinely worked in this area, the ladies not having quite the same perceived dangerousness to men as the male patients have to women. So many of the mentally ill have relationship problems with the opposite sex, and safe environments to address these issues have long been overdue.

The positive result of this is that relationships are developed that are often very beneficial. Conversely, however, try placing a female patient in a regional secure unit amongst ten ill men and telling her that she is in a therapeutic environment!

Primary nursing

This works well if the nurses are skilled and really interested in what they are doing. In most cases, however, primary nursing is viewed as a 'paper exercise'. Good primary nursing, in my experience, has many benefits. It improves a patient's lifestyle, and a partnership is formed in which patients have some control over their own lives and are actively encouraged to make decisions and take responsibility for themselves.

A good nurse working alongside a patient can trigger as much healing as the highest trained psychotherapist. It is about being there, relating and showing compassion on a consistent basis. Do not underestimate the effect you can have on your patients by showing a sincere interest – or indeed the opposite!

Partnerships in care

To empower users has, on the whole, a very positive effect in giving people a voice, a platform where what they say has value and they are not just some mentally ill person. To be heard and listened to is, in itself, a form of therapy; in being part of effecting positive change, it is very validating.

Nursing ethos

Changes being introduced to phase out or retrain what are known in Broadmoor circles as 'Dinosaurs', and the methods they inherited, have led to an improved service. No longer the tyranny of the vast majority of charge nurses brought up with the old school who shouted and you jumped. The mellowing out of the regime, the introduction of new blood, of liberal people, is of the highest benefit. I have seen the whole atmosphere change: from a ward surging with very damaging undercurrents to one where life was that much more receptive to growth. The restructuring that led to ward managers and team leaders replacing the old charge nurses has led to more democracy. That these people leaders are carefully chosen is of the utmost importance.

Drama

Drama has, since Ancient Greek times, been appreciated as being therapeutic. To see life portrayed with all its many facets – from joy to tragedy – has great benefits. When the Royal Shakespeare Company came to Broadmoor in 1989 to perform Hamlet, the effect was profound. The play deals with madness, murder and suicide, all matters that have touched people in Broadmoor. That a book was written off the back of that performance (Cox, 1992), and a couple of others since, is testament to its strong impact.

The Geese Theatre Company, who were set up for purely thera-peutic reasons and who work in custodial settings, also came in from time to time. Their week spent working exclusively on one ward was, for the patients I spoke to, worth a year's normal group therapy. One did not know how he could ever go back to facing the routine, boring groups after such a dynamic experience. Indeed, months afterwards, the participants were all still working through the effects of that week. There was a drama therapy project in which I took part, the resulting growth in confidence and sense of common purpose being very enjoyable.

There are so many creative art forms that are beginning to be more focused in Broadmoor, music and art therapy being just two. Being creative – playing as adults – has been valuable for people who may have played precious little as children. They can be more relaxed, learn to work together and express things that are safer or easier to express with the end of a drumstick or the sweep of a brush.

The Snoezelen Rompa room

Imported from Holland, the Snoezelen room is installed on two female wards in Broadmoor. It is a comforting room where a patient can get away from the ward and be in control of whatever sensory inputs she likes, for example music, lighting, gentle vibration or tactile sensations. It is a safe place and, on a crowded and disturbed ward, gives people that space to be at peace in place of self-seclusion. It is very popular on the wards and is part of many patients' treatment plans. Aromatherapy is also now available on some wards.

There has been a profound shift in the way of dealing with self-harm by the use of 'specialling' (when nurses closely monitor the patient). Less punitive methods and attitudes on the part of nurses are also leading to patients coming forward to discuss matters of concern and to trust nurses more.

Complaints procedure

The complaints procedure has made great advances. It is vitally important that patients can complain, and improved procedures are giving patients more confidence that they may be believed and that there is some protection against abuse. Once again, this gives the patient some power (even if it is often not used in the most appropriate ways). Nurses do not like being complained about – nobody does – but how else do we learn if not from mistakes? 'The nurse is always right' is now less in evidence, thank goodness. This also encourages nurses to think of more creative solutions to problems than simply enforcing their will.

These have been some of the improvements in my time. Now let us consider how services could be improved from the point of view of users.

The skill base of the forensic nurse

I will start with what I believe is the most profound improvement that can be made, and that is in the range of skills of the forensic nurse. Forensic nurses are the ones who deliver the service and who, to a great extent, make or break it. It is crucial for nurses, to enable them to meet individual needs, that their skill base is diversified. People are unique, their problems multifaceted, needing to be addressed in an appropriate way - which is often not possible because the skills just do not seem to be there.

Allow me to be more specific. Grief and bereavement are, in our society, taboo subjects (as is, to a lesser extent, sexuality). Many people just do not know how to react to a bereaved person. That this extends within the forensic setting is only natural, but very unhealthy. In the world of Broadmoor, people who have killed loved ones are – as the reader will appreciate – very common, but there has been precious little work carried out by psychiatrists and nurses alike to address the bereavement issues of these patients. This situation is, of course, one extreme; there are also the more natural deaths of loved ones as well as losses that are often totally ignored – loss of health, loss of sanity, loss of trust, loss of freedom, loss of career, loss of dignity ... I could go on and on.

These are things that are important for discussion as they are live issues for patients. There is a need for a specialist post at Broadmoor, which hopefully has now been realised. I am sure there is also the need for an appraisal of the nature of people's losses in less secure settings and a need for specific training to be more sensitive to this.

I began with counselling skills, and these are important whether you believe in concentrating on people's positive attributes and life chances, or in working from a deeper viewpoint. We need people to hear us, and that means with both ear and brain connected. This is something that is often amiss on overstretched wards but needs to be worked at very hard in order to achieve success. Nurses specialising in counselling skills in issues of sexuality, race and culture, family therapy, addiction and specific types of offending are needed. There is no harm in overlapping skills in talking treatments as this area is consistently underfunded. There is also the opportunity for the nurse to use and learn about other skills such as the arts in order to facilitate communication and expression.

I believe that a lot of staff need further training to enable them to work in a more positive and reflective way. Nurses themselves can be prejudiced, whether it is in the area of race, sexuality, or offending behaviour. That prejudice finds its way into care networks is not at all surprising, but this needs to be challenged, and for this there is a requirement for better training.

Loving relationships

Loving relationships between patients are often seen in a negative light. The reader may already have encountered this: two ill people, for example, making a pact for life only for it to break up shortly afterwards. Many staff think that patients should not be allowed to marry in Broadmoor. However, each case must be seen on its own merits. There are problems in big institutions, where a couple's needs are not really accommodated, and also in smaller hospitals, where they are seen as counterproductive to treatment. Such areas are highly controversial with both patients and nurses.

People in relationships should be treated with respect and given the time and space to make their own mistakes – if that is what will

happen – or indeed successes. So much can be learnt from relationships with people who have found problems within relationships in the
past. A skilled and knowledgeable effort to work with, rather than
against, those relationships needs to be found. I am heavily influenced
by my experience of Broadmoor, where there is still great opposition to
relationships. I am talking here in the main about male–female relationships, but gay patients, especially male ones, are a subject of some
controversy. The thought of patients being given privacy is unthink-
able to most and, some would say, unworkable in Broadmoor.

However, on the subject of patients who have partners outside,
there should be the opportunity for conjugal visits – the patients are
in hospital after all. Of course, it is this sort of topic that the media
industry takes much salacious interest in and hence negatively influences politicians.

Equal opportunities

There is currently a special focus on equal opportunities in the NHS,
but what does this mean to the individual nurse? The ethnic make-
up of the average forensic client group needs this focus. Treatment
plans need to be drawn up with an awareness of people's differing
cultural needs. Treating people equally does not mean that one
treats them the same.

Medication

In my time, a wide gap has existed with regard to explanations of the
use of psychiatric drugs, including their side-effects. It is important to
note that, in France, instead of prescribing medications such as
procyclidine and orphenadrine to counteract the side-effects of
antipsychotic drugs, physicians use vitamins (National Schizophrenic Fellowship, 1994). Given the side-effects of certain medications (namely tardive dyskinesia), one can wonder why this method
has not been at least tried in the UK. A better explanation and
discussion of drugs is important to empower users. A good understanding of the drugs and their side-effects should not, because of
arousing uncomfortable feelings in nurses (and psychiatrists), lead to
silence, as it does most of the time.

User groups

The continuing involvement of user-led groups in the discussion of
provision of services is very important. It is important for nurses to

keep on listening. Hopefully, this development will not be reversed as there are quite a few in the user movement who make good trainers and communicators.

The lazy nurse

As an important consideration, I ask for the measurement of nurses' work. For too long the lazy have prospered, consistently putting computer games and television before patients' interests. Fixed-term contracts may provide the shake-up that the less well-intentioned need for a better service. This should not, however, present any fear for those nurses who are committed to their patients. Such strategies are particularly needed in the larger institutions where, from experience, people hide, although all around them needs are waiting to be met. This may address the apathy and lack of productivity of certain individuals.

Finally, a personal message. Nurses probably all have differing personal reasons for coming into nursing (some possibly entering 'the side door to the hospital' with problems similar to those of existing patients). But there is primarily a desire to help out in some way. For some, this is much easier than for others. We all find out what we like to do, and if it helps others, so much the better. It is quite possible however to be counterproductive because of reasons such as carrying one's own 'baggage' to work.

When you go into work next month having been up all night with your youngest child, when your partner is behaving like a Neanderthal, when, having been relieved to find that the sun is actually shining, you relax and enter the unit, only to be met by three patients screaming at each other, it is then that the test of your mettle begins.

But spare a thought - you'll probably need counselling too! They say that there is one in every family and *it's true*: we have a psychiatric nurse in ours. One of the things that I and she have discussed is how, for example, it is often the patient who has to act sane and help the nurse who is carrying his or her personality problem into everyday interactions on the ward. With this in mind, isn't it fair to apply a few home truths?

What is being asked of me? Presumably, apart from flogging myself for the prison officer nurses, the implicit understanding is that I need to grow and adapt to the situation in which I find myself.

If it's what I have to do, why not you? To meet each new hurdle, to cope with the boredom, the abuse and whatever mental gymnastics are going on in your own backyard, you need to grow. The challenge is to get people on the healthier rails of life. Training is fine, but you have to work through the nitty-gritty, the personal relationships that are fraught with so much distrust and fear. To put someone else first, before your emotions, before your own clamouring needs, is not easy. You have to work on yourself.

Finally, it is 'normal' for human beings to be prejudiced and ignorant to some extent. With this in mind, I would like to finish with the words of a solicitor – Lucy Scott-Moncrieff – who has extensive experience of representing patients at Broadmoor:

> ... people are going to have likes and dislikes, this is human nature. I think it's a pity that likes and dislikes sometimes have to be disguised behind a jargon of professionalism when you might simply say that you can't stand the person. I've never believed in objectivity. Human beings are not objective. The thing to do is to try and be aware of your subjectivity; not allow it to get in the way too much but not to pretend it doesn't exist.

References

Cox M (Ed.) (1992) Shakespeare Comes to Broadmoor. London: Jessica Kingsley.
National Schizophrenic Fellowship (1994) National Schizophrenic Fellowship Newsletter (Winter): 5.
The Chronicle (1994) Broadmoor Community Magazine. Interview with Solicitor, Lucy Scott-Moncrieff. (June/July edition).

Chapter 9
Empowerment of mentally disordered offenders within a controlled environment

NEIL KITCHINER

This chapter will present an analysis of empowerment within a controlled environment. It is intended to examine the attributes and characteristics of this concept and will relate these to the empowerment of the forensic patient in a controlled setting. Wilson's (1963) strategy for this concept analysis is used to facilitate the process.

The aim of this concept analysis is to gain a better understanding of how nurses try to empower the patients with whom they work. It is intended that this process will highlight the particular attributes of empowerment and that this will assist nurses and other mental health workers to promote this valuable concept effectively within their working environment.

Empowerment within the nursing literature

The Collins *Thesaurus* defines the term 'empower' as to 'allow, authorize, delegate, enable, permit, qualify, sanction'. The suffix '-ment' can be defined as 'a result or product, the act, fact or process of art' (Guralnik, 1970). The definitions that have been developed and used in the nursing literature do not always describe the concept itself but reflect the populations being studied. Hawks (1992) and Clifford (1993) both make reference to empowerment in relation to nurse education. Hawks defines empowerment as the 'interpersonal process of providing the proper tools, resources and environment to build, develop and increase the ability and effectiveness of others to set and reach goals for individual ends'. Clifford's (1993) study raised questions of whether nurse teachers have the necessary resources and tools to empower nurses in this way.

A study by Thomas (1992), which considered the quality of life of elderly people on dialysis, argued for nurses to be educated to accept the concept of patient empowerment, but gave no indication of the type of education needed to achieve this.

Gibson (1991) and Jones and Meleis (1993) conceptualise empowerment as referring to people's – both nurses' and patients' – attributes, which would include individual rights, strengths and abilities. Others have suggested that there may be a tension between the concepts of caring and empowerment, and that nurses must maximise patients' independence and minimise their dependence by creating a partnership between nurse and patient in which the nurse puts her skills and knowledge at the disposal of the patient, whom she trusts to make responsible decisions (Malin and Teasdale, 1991). Although admirable, this view does not take into account the requirements of those patients who, because of illness, are unable to make responsible decisions.

It could be argued that the consumer movement has, at its core, a desire to empower individuals with rights of information, a say in how *experts* design and run services, and freedom to choose where and when services (or health care treatment) are used (Malin, 1990). This, however, does not take into account the less able, disadvantaged, oppressed individual who may need support to make an informed decision. Allmark and Klarzynski (1992), whilst arguing against nurse advocacy, suggest that nurses who support the empowerment of patients should be developing independent advocacy systems and demanding legal changes. Unfortunately, Allmark and Klarzynski do not indicate how these changes will empower the patients they are intended to.

Empowerment within a controlled environment

Controlled environments are specially designated facilities set up for the MDO patient population. To be deemed eligible for admission to such a facility, two criteria must be met: the patient must exhibit a mental disorder requiring compulsory treatment, and he or she must present a risk of being dangerous, violent or having criminal propensity. Controlled environments foster a health care regime coupled with security restrictions placed upon patients, and will be either a maximum security Special Hospital or an MSU (Burrow, 1993a). Because of the criminal and/or dangerous propensities indicated by these patients' past behaviour, their health management involves a control of the interpersonal and physical environment through necessary security operations and monitoring of the potential for future dangerousness (Burrow, 1993b). This emphasis on maintaining control has implications for nursing practice.

Bernier (1986) and Burrow (1993c) argue that the themes of security, detention and punishment of the criminal justice system often clash with the goal of improvement or maintenance of mental health, commonly referred to as the therapy versus custody debate. These authors ask whether it is possible to provide individualised, patient-centred, health-promoting care while confining patients – often for many years and sometimes without a clear treatment programme – to ensure the protection of the public. Studies that have surveyed forensic nursing have indicated that forensic patients have unique characteristics that impact on the treatment environment and the provision of nursing care (Phillips, 1983). These characteristics have been documented by Hammond (1983) and Burrow (1992) within patients who display daily aggressive, self-destructive (self-mutilatory) and property-damaging behaviours. These challenging behaviours often create a gulf between patients and staff, at the same time dictating the atmosphere felt by both parties on the ward.

Goffman (1961) argues that the moral climate is often seen differently by nurses and patients. Nurses may feel that they are emphasising psychiatric care in therapeutic environments when they use interventions such as privilege systems, seclusion and restraint, and medication. Patients often perceive these same interventions as humiliating, punishment or forced containment. In response to this, Hendry (1983), a Special Hospital Chief Nursing Officer, argued for a normalisation of the patients' day, an alternative means of assisting patients to progress through the hospital and a greater emphasis on therapeutic participation rather than security-consciousness.

A study by Fogel and Martin (1992) looking at the mental health of incarcerated women found a high prevalence of mental health problems. They advocated that nurses should aim to increase the degree and quality of maternal–child contact during incarceration and the setting-up of self-help groups, counselling, stress management and self-esteem enhancement work for women inmates. Within the secure hospital environments, there are rehabilitative resources for patients – educational, social, occupational, recreational and remedial – that may be used to help in the empowerment of the patient group in order to make them ready for their transfers.

Unfortunately, studies have indicated that there has been poor success in securing the resocialisation, rehabilitative and employment skills of forensic patients from these environments (Norris, 1984).

Other related concepts

Roberts (1983) and Freire (1971) have written about various oppressed groups within our society, including negros, Jews and women. I would suggest that psychiatric patients should be added to this list. Freire has identified the major characteristics of oppressing behaviour as the ability of dominant groups to identify their norms and values as the right ones in a society, and the utilisation of an initial power base to enforce them. In most cases of oppression, the dominant group looks and acts differently from the subordinate group. Roberts makes reference to the 'submissive aggression syndrome' in which the oppressed person may feel aggressive towards the oppressor but is unable to express this directly. Hence aggression may be directed internally or in a self-destructive way.

This submissive aggression syndrome may be used to analyse how nurses in controlled environments use the moral and legal codes of society to enforce their norms and detain the forensic patient. The nurses are distinguishable from the patient group by their uniform and the obvious carrying of keys. Patients' aggression and self-harming behaviours are viewed by the nurses as symptoms of mental illness yet, according to the submissive aggression syndrome, these would be usual behaviours for oppressed groups.

Women with mental health problems are also an oppressed group. This is evident as they are often put in particularly powerless positions, most mental health services failing to acknowledge their unique needs and rights. They are often unable to make best use of services because they cannot bring along their children, and they are seldom given the choice of a female psychiatrist or therapist (Read and Wallcraft, 1992).

Miller and Biley (1992) highlight the feminist movement as a group concerned with fighting oppression, particularly the use of power by one group to dominate another. These authors do so by rejecting this repressive form of power and advocating instead personal empowerment, the application of personal power promotion, transformation, justice and peace. The ideals proposed by the feminist movement could provide a useful starting point for forensic nurses to re-evaluate their own practice when attempting to empower their patients. Kendall (1992) urges nurses to break away from their preoccupation with adaptation and coping in order to become leaders in the struggle for emancipation from the oppressive forces by which many patients are bound.

The concept of control also has a role in this discussion believed that to be in control of one's life is both desirabl healthy yet the patient is assumed to take a passively dependent posture in many if not all health care interactions (Bloom and Wilson, 1972). Nursing, like so many other professions, has been successful in obtaining institutional powers that set limits on patient freedoms and powers (Reeder, 1972). The idea of control has been articulated in the work of Frankl (1963) and Antonovsky (1972). They emphasise individual choice, making decisions and actively creating meaning in one's life, with the feeling that events are comprehensible rather than bewildering and are under some kind of control.

Others have argued that this is not true for all individuals and that some patients may want relief from decision-making and the burden of autonomy (O'Neil, 1984). Some may not wish to be involved in decisions concerning their own treatment (Lancaster, 1982). Researchers have demonstrated that having control over aversive events is preferred by subjects and that control has beneficial effects such as the reduction of anxiety and fewer distressing complications (Wilson-Barnett and Fordham, 1982). Studies have also shown that fewer situational (institutional) constraints are associated with higher levels of life satisfaction, alertness and adjustment. The manner in which the patient perceives control in daily activities is expected to influence his or her sense of well-being (Chang, 1978).

People who believe that they have control over their lives are said to have an internal locus of control. Those who believe that they have no control over the events in their lives, these being due to chance, fate, the system or whatever, are classified as having an external locus of control (Chang, 1980). Chang's hypothesis of the external locus of control could be successfully applied to the forensic psychiatric patient. Others in powerful positions make decisions on all aspects of his or her life, often with little or no collaboration or consultation taking place to elicit the individual's views or wishes.

Antecedents to empowerment

Hawks (1992) maintains that the environment for empowerment needs to be one of nurturing and caring, in which several conditions, including trust, openness, honesty, genuineness and communication, must exist coupled with an acceptance of people as individuals with mutual respect, value for others, courtesy and shared vision between patient and nurse (Table 9.1). Health care professionals cannot empower people: only people can empower themselves. However, nurses can help patients to develop, secure and use resources that will promote or foster a sense of control and self-efficacy (Gibson, 1991).

Table 9.1. Attributes of empowerment and controlled environments

Functional attributes of empowerment	Controlled environments and empowerment
Interpersonal process of relationship-building	Staff maintain distance Patient–staff gap
Open communication Goal-setting together	Poor communication Patients often have no understanding of treatment plan
Development of potential Aim to maximise independence	Blanket, unindividualised care Institutionalisation
Patient encouraged to make choices	Lack of choices as a result of security operations
Patients seen as deserving basic human rights	Patients seen as dangerous offenders in need of control
Patients free to express their innermost feelings without fear of misinterpretation or punishment for doing so	Patients feel they have to act in a certain way to secure transfer
Patients control their circumstances, as beneficial, healthy	Nurses have institutional powers and set limits on patient freedom
The fewer the situational constraints, the higher the levels of expressed patient satisfaction	Patients live in locked, controlled environments where parole, searches, cameras and high walls are prominent features

Health care professionals need to surrender the need for control and adopt the stance necessary for co-operation. Haney (1988) believes that the patient's capacity for growth and self-determination needs to be respected. Individuals have the ability to make decisions and act on their own behalf, although they may need information and help to do so.

Empowerment is seen as a collaborative process (Wallerstein and Bernstein, 1988) between the nurse and patient. Thus, the nurse is challenged to expose any power imbalances that prohibit people from achieving their full potential. This would involve giving patients as much power and control as possible to enable decision-making, based upon timely and accurate information, regarding their own unique health care needs.

Consequences of empowerment

Nurses need to turn their attention to the conditions that control, influence and produce health or illness in human beings. Forensic nurses should therefore seek out any rituals, attitudes and practices that hinder the empowerment process and develop those which promote it. Nurses should strive to become more self-aware, recognise the powerful position they hold as a result of their knowledge and expertise, and make it available as a tool for the empowerment of the patient (Katz, 1984).

The health care professional needs a commitment to serve rather than to accumulate power for personal use (Gibson, 1991). Forensic nurses could best serve the wider society that they protect by empowering the forensic patients for whom they care to achieve optimum functioning. In part, this will be achieved by supplying patients with the necessary information and skills development opportunities to survive in the community upon discharge with an enabled internal locus of control. As a result of this process, the empowered person will possess an increased ability to set and reach goals for individual and social ends (Hawks, 1992).

In the forensic setting, this may be mediated within services that aim to support people in crisis to regain a sense of being in charge of their lives by encouraging them to take an active and positive role in their treatment, with full information about different treatments, how they work and possible drawbacks (Read and Wallcraft, 1992).

A staff group who are not afraid to get interpersonally involved with patients during their hospitalisation, and who actively encourage patients to be creative, assertive and strong, are required to deliver this type of service. Read and Wallcraft's (1992) recommendations suggest that staff should adhere to the following criteria when trying to empower service users:

- let patients know their rights;
- ask patients what they want from the service;
- recognise patients' talents, capabilities and potential;
- give as much information as patients can assimilate about the drugs prescribed, the patients' diagnoses and the options open to them;
- above all, talk to the patients.

Empowerment redefined

Empowerment may be redefined as a process of helping the patient to assert control over the factors that affect his or her life in an environment that treats the person as a unique individual with rights to respect and dignity. The process of promoting and enhancing the individual's abilities to meet personal needs involves helping the person to develop a critical awareness of the situation and facilitating the emergence of a joint realistic plan of action (Gibson, 1991). The nurse serves as a resource mobiliser and advocate so that the patient can have access to the resources required. The success of the required outcomes must be defined by both patient and nurse. Empowerment may then be viewed as a combination of personal choice and social responsibility in health care (Minkler, 1989) (Boxes 9.1 and 9.2).

Research into this concept and activity of empowerment might usefully concentrate on the following patient outcomes: self-efficacy, sense of control, growth, and improved health and well-being

---

Box 9.1. An empowered service user

Patient X is a young man, sent to a Special Hospital within an offence of manslaughter while severely psychotic:

I was transferred to a maximum security hospital via prison. On my arrival I felt like I was on the bottom rung of the ladder of life – not deserving any respect, without any power, not sure that I deserved to be alive after the terrible crime I had committed.

From the first day the nurses started to reassure me that I was safe, and encouraged me to be open and honest with them, to share my feelings and problems, so together we could plan my treatment, giving me the feeling that they cared about me.

The staff encouraged and accommodated my regular family visits whilst continually reassuring me that they would help me overcome my illness, with the aim of transferring me to a medium secure unit. Once stable and over hearing voices I was able to start attending the hospital workshops, education classes, and recreational facilities where an individualised daily programme was negotiated with me, with the aim of increasing my self-confidence, trust, and self-respect. By the time I was ready to be transferred to a medium secure unit I had dealt with many of my problems and received education about my illness. I had obtained a certificate in sports and recreational instruction which helped me to obtain a responsible 'job of trust' in the hospital gym, devising physical programmes for other patients.

On the ward, I was instrumental in fund raising activities to buy new furniture, paint and wallpaper, and helped organise its redecoration. I was also active on the Patients' Council within the hospital to help bring about change on behalf of my peers. From day one of my stay in that hospital I felt staff were interested in helping me deal with my offence and the symptoms of my illness, encouraging me to take an active part in my recovery and treatment.

Box 9.2. An disempowered service user

On arrival at the maximum security hospital I felt alone and afraid within this alien environment. The nurses were unapproachable and seemed uninterested in me as in individual; they were more concerned with following me around the ward until I was locked in my bedroom for the night. Even when I received my weekly visits from my family the staff were always within earshot watching me.

Once I had regained some control of my senses through the help of medication I felt like my life was going nowhere, the days dragged due to the boredom of the sterile ward routine. No one was interested in me as a person or helping me to move on to a less secure environment. Professionals would visit me without any explanation as to how they could help me and would then disappear for weeks on end. I felt that I had no say in my care or my future, my life was in the hands of strangers who seemed unconcerned about my views or wishes. I felt powerless and unable to control any part of my life.

(Gibson, 1991). Although no single measure can adequately capture this concept, Rappaport (1984), whilst acknowledging the difficulty in measuring empowerment, adds that each attempt at measurement, intervention and description in a particular context adds to the understanding of this useful construct.

The primary consideration

Brandon (1991) insisted that people for whom services are designed and presented should always be in the forefront of health care thinking. People are the primary consideration: what are their needs, what do they want, and how do professionals and people together achieve this? This point is developed further by Bynoe (1992) when discussing the forensic patient. He advocates the formulation of fundamental standards, rights and expectations recognising that those having to use the service, and detained in it against their will, are citizens as well as users of health and social services, and that their rights as citizens need to be clearly understood and acknowledged as much as their expectations as users of a health service. In short, he argued for people detained in hospitals to be viewed as citizens first and patients second.

Conclusions

This analysis of the concept of empowerment within a controlled environment has many implications for nursing practice, the patients' environment and relationships between health care professionals and patients to be empowered, as well as research and education.

If this concept is truly promoted by forensic nurses as service providers who adhere to the principles outlined in this paper, they may achieve more success in raising the profile of this doubly stigmatised group of patients and better prepare them for life in the community or at least in conditions of lesser security.

References

Allmark P, Klarzynski R (1992) The case against nurse advocacy. British Journal of Nursing 2(1): 33–7.

Antonovsky A (1972) Breakdown: a needed fourth step in the conceptual armamentarium of modern medicine. Social Science and Medicine 6: 537–44.

Bernier SL (1986) Corrections and mental health. Journal of Psychosocial Health 24(6): 20–5.

Bloom S, Wilson R (1972) Patient–practioner relationships. In Freeman H et al (Eds) Handbook of Medical Sociology, 2nd Edn. Englewood Cliffs, NJ: Prentice-Hall.

Brandon D (1991) User power. In Barker PJ, Baldwin S (Eds) Ethical Issues in Mental Health. London: Chapman & Hall.

Burrow S (1992) The deliberate self-harming behaviour of patients within a British special hospital. Journal of Advanced Nursing 17: 138–48.

Burrow S (1993a) The contribution of secure hospitals to social control. British Journal of Nursing 12(18): 891.

Burrow S (1993b) An outline of the forensic nursing role. British Journal of Nursing 12(18): 899–905.

Burrow S (1993c) The treatment and security needs of special hospital patient: nursing perspective. Journal of Advanced Nursing 18: 1267–78.

Bynoe I (1992) Treatment, Care and Security: Waiting for Change. London: MIND.

Chang BL (1978) Generalized expectancy, situational perception, and morale among institutionalized aged. Nursing Research 27(5): 316–24.

Chang BL (1980) Black and white elderly: morale and perception of control. Western Journal of Nursing Research 2(1): 371–92.

Clifford C (1993) The role of the nurse teachers in the empowerment of nurses through research. Nurse Education Today 13: 47–54.

Fogel CI, Martin SL (1992) The mental health of incarcerated women. Western Journal of Nursing Research 14(1): 30–40.

Frankl VE (1963) Man's Search for Meaning. New York: Pocket Books.

Freire P (1971) Pedagogy of the Oppressed. New York: Herder & Herder.

Gibson CH (1991) A concept analysis of empowerment. Journal of Advanced Nursing 16: 354–61.

Goffman E (1961) Asylums. Chicago: Aldine.

Guralnik D (1970) Websters New World Dictionary of the American Language, 2nd Colour Edn. New York: The World.

Hammond J (1983) Behaviour modification at Rampton hospital. Nursing Times 79(39):49-52.

Haney P (1988) Providing empowerment to the person with AIDS. Social Work 33(3): 251–6.

Hawks JH (1992) Empowerment in nursing education: concept analysis and application to philosophy, learning and instruction. Journal of Advanced Nursing 17: 609–18.

Hendry M (1983) Nursing behind bars. Nursing Mirror 15(9): 16–18.

Jones PS, Meleis AI (1993) Health is empowerment. Advances in Nursing Science 15(3): 1–14.

Katz R (1984) Empowerment and synergy: expanding the community's healing resources. Prevention in Human Services 3: 201–26.

Kendall J (1992) Fighting back: promoting emancipatory nursing actions. Advances in Nursing Science 15(2): 1–15.

Lancaster W (1982) Health care marketing: a model for planning change. In Lancaster J, Lancaster W (Ed) Concepts for Advanced Nursing Practice: the Nurse as a Change Agent. St Louis: C V Mosby.

Malin N (1990) Normalisation and Community Care Policy. Paper given at the International Conference on Family Policies in Europe. Alcide de Gasperi, Bologna, Italy, 16–18 January.

Malin N, Teasdale K (1991) Caring versus empowerment: considerations for nursing practice. Journal of Advanced Nursing 16: 657–62.

Miller B, Biley F (1992) An exploration of issues relating to feminism and nurse education. Nurse Education Today 12: 274–8.

Minkler M (1989) Health education, health promotion and the open society: an historical perspective. Health Education Quarterly 16(1): 17–30.

Norris M (1984) Integration of special hospital patients into the community. Aldershot: Gower.

O'Neil O (1984) Paternalism and partial autonomy. Journal of Medical Ethics 10: 173–8.

Phillips MS (1983) Forensic psychiatry: nurses' attitudes revealed. Dimensions in Health Service 60(9): 41–3.

Rappaport J (1984) Studies in empowerment: introduction to the issue. Prevention in Human Services 3: 1–7.

Read J, Wallcraft J (1992) Guidelines for Empowering Users of Mental Health Services. London: Confederation of Health Service Employees/MIND.

Reeder LG (1972) The patient-client as a consumer: some observations on the changing professional–client relationship. Journal of Health and Social Behaviour 13: 406–12.

Roberts SJ (1983) Oppressed group behaviour: implications for nursing. Advances in Nursing Science (Jul): 21–30.

Thomas N (1992) Measurement of quality of life for elderly people on dialysis. British Journal of Nursing 1(6): 281–5.

Wallerstein N, Bernstein E (1988) Empowerment education: Freire's ideas adapted to health education. Health Education Quarterly 15(4): 379–94.

Wilson J (1963) Thinking with Concepts. London: Cambridge University Press.

Wilson-Barnett J, Fordham M (1982) Recovery from Illness. Chichester: John Wiley & Sons.

Chapter 10
Criminal responsibility and mental illness

FRANK HANILY

A long-standing principle of English criminal law is to be found in the common law maxim *actus non facit reum nisi mens sit rea* (an act does not make a man guilty of a crime unless his mind is also guilty). It follows that the prosecution must prove both that the accused had caused the event or that responsibility is to be attributed to him for having broken the law (*actus reus*), and that he had it in mind to cause the event or to bring about the state of affairs that led to the law being broken (*mens rea*). The burden of proof lies with the prosecution to prove beyond reasonable doubt that the defendant committed the crime (*Wolmington* v. *Director of Public Prosecutions*, 1935). The jury must acquit the defendant (even though they are not fully satisfied that the defendant's story is true) unless they are satisfied beyond reasonable doubt that the defendant's story is untrue. This rule is generally applied but with one exception at common law – the defence of insanity (Smith and Hogan, 1992).

However, there is a tension between legal and medical professionals. Legal powers have been used to counteract what have been viewed as shortcomings in medical management, and vice versa when the legal approach was seen to have failed. The purpose of this chapter is to show how mental illness operates as mitigation in criminal proceedings. This account will chart the early development of this defence and explore how it has evolved over the years as knowledge and awareness of mental health matters expanded. Issues such as the scope of the defence and diminished responsibility will be explained and illustrated using case law.

The origins of the insanity defence

In the eighteenth and nineteenth centuries, the judiciary made various attempts to define 'criminal insanity'. In 1724, Edward Arnold was charged with attempting to murder Lord Onslow. Arnold had a belief that Lord Onslow would enter his body and torment him. The trial judge, Justice Tracy, gave the following instruction on what was necessary for a person to be acquitted of a serious offence on grounds of insanity:

> Totally deprived of his understanding and memory and does not know what he is doing, no more than an infant, a brute, or a wild beast, such a one is never the object of punishment. (Walker, 1967)

This became known as the 'wild beast test'. Fortunately, after an appeal, the accused was spared from the hangman's noose.

The concept of criminal responsibility developed slowly, as indeed did the understanding and treatment of insanity over the centuries. However, the nineteenth century saw several major trials that resulted in important guidelines for determining the criminal responsibility of the insane. The case concerning Hadfield, who shot at King George III at Drury Lane, London in 1800, highlighted the inadequacy of the law as it stood and pointed the way towards improvement. Hadfield had suffered head injuries in the wars of 1796 and had been discharged from the army on grounds of insanity. His delusional beliefs led to his attempting to kill the King in the knowledge that this would be punishable by death. Hadfield's successful defence was that:

> if a man is labouring under a delusion if you are satisfied that the delusion existed at the time of the offence and that the act was done under its influence, then he cannot be considered as guilty of any crime.

During the trial, it was clear that Hadfield had been able to distinguish right from wrong and fully comprehended the nature of the alleged crime, so the verdict was fraught with judicial anomalies and difficulties. Hadfield obviously posed a threat to himself and to others, and it was essential that he be detained despite the fact that his detention would be illegal. As a consequence, the Criminal Lunatics Act 1800 was passed and made retrospective. This change in the law obliged the court, when a person was found insane, to order his safe custody in some suitable place 'until His Majesty's Pleasure be known'.

The precedent set in the Hadfield case was by no means the rule. In 1812, Bellingham shot the Prime Minister and was tried and executed within 1 week even though he suffered from a paranoid and deluded state. However, in Oxford's case in 1840, the defendant was found not guilty of attempted murder on the basis of insanity, as the jury was instructed that:

> A person may commit a criminal act and not be responsible. If some contributory disease was in truth the acting power within him, which he could not resist, he would not be responsible.

The current definition of criminal insanity arose following the case of McNaughten in 1843. He suffered from a delusion that the Tory Party was persecuting him and shot the Prime Minister's Private Secretary. His acquittal on grounds of insanity caused public outcry, but the 'McNaughten Rules' have remained the cornerstone of the criminal insanity defence in Britain, Canada and the USA. These rules state that:

> at the time of the act, he [the defendant] was labouring under such a defect of reason, from disease of the mind, that he did not know the nature and quality of his act; or if he did know it, he did not know that what he was doing was wrong.

These Rules involves two disciplines – law and psychiatry – and they have two functions that need to be clearly distinguished. The first is to provide criteria for excusing the mentally disordered from criminal liability on the basis that the insanity negates *mens rea*. The second function is to enable a psychiatric disposal (Grubin, 1991). In practice, the defence is used in only the gravest of offences: 'Its moribund state, with only one or two gasps a year, may not worry Judges and Psychiatrists ... but it should worry those who want to see mentally disordered offenders disposed of' (Hamilton, 1986; Walker, 1981). Despite this view, the Rules still have great importance because they remain the legal test of criminal responsibility and because they set a limit to the defences of automatism and, in theory, diminished responsibility (Smith and Hogan, 1992).

Development of services and legislation

Whilst the courts were recognising and acknowledging the criminally insane, the processes of dealing with and treating this group after disposal were much slower in developing. Broadmoor Hospital, the first institution for criminal lunatics, was born out of the accumulation of large numbers of people found insane following the Criminal Lunatics Act 1800. The Trial of Lunatics Act 1883 led to a change in the verdict from 'not guilty by reason of insanity' to 'guilty but insane', which continued until the former was restored in the

Criminal Procedures (Insanity) Act 1964. The Mental Health Act 1959 opened up the asylums; as a result, mentally ill people were able to receive treatment in the community and a series of government reports made new recommendations for provisions for MDOs (Department of Health, 1961; Department of Health and Social Security, 1974; Home Office, 1964).

However, it was not until after the case of Graham Young in 1972 that a political impetus for change occurred. The Butler Committee (Department of Health and Social Security and Home Office, 1975) undertook a fundamental review of services and provision, a consequence of which was that more resources were made available to provide care. More recently, the Reed Review (Department of Health and Home Office, 1992) examined the services available for MDOs in the community, hospitals and prisons. The Woolf Report (Home Office, 1991) into prison disturbances during 1990 recommended that the number of MDOs in the penal system should be minimised. Following this, court diversion schemes were developed to identify and divert MDOs from custody.

Defendants found unfit to plead or under a disability by the courts

The issue of the defendant's sanity can be raised at any time during the criminal process. The legal test relating to unfitness to plead was laid down in the case of *R* v. *Pritchard* in 1836. Pritchard was charged with bestiality but did not plead to the accusation; a jury was empanelled and found that he was deaf and mute by visitation – but it was also established that he could read and write. The court stated that the accused should be 'of sufficient intellect to comprehend the course of the proceedings in the trial so as to make a proper defence, to challenge a juror to whom he might wish to object and comprehend the details of the evidence'. In essence, there appear to be five basic criteria to be satisfied when fitness to plead is at issue, these being:

- knowing the difference between the pleas of 'guilty' and 'not guilty';
- being able to understand the details of the evidence;
- having the ability to follow court proceedings;
- knowing that a juror can be challenged;
- being able to instruct legal advisers.

Fitness to plead is decided by a jury usually, but not necessarily, after the presentation of psychiatric evidence (Mitchell and Richardson, 1985). Once found unfit to plead, an individual is dealt with under Section 5A of the Criminal Procedure (Insanity and Unfitness to Plead) Act 1991 (which amended the Criminal Procedures (Insanity) Act 1964), where the finding is referred to as 'disability in bar of trial'. The 1964 Act was widely criticised, largely because of its inflexibility in the disposal of offenders and the lack of opportunity to hold a 'trial of the facts' (Mackay, 1991). Under the 1964 Act, the only disposal available to the courts, on a finding of unfitness to plead, was the equivalent of a combination of Sections 37 and 41 of the Mental Health Act 1983 – a hospital order with restrictions, without limit of time.

White (1992), in critiquing the 1991 Act, remarked that there were two main changes, the first of which related to the procedure to be followed when doubts were raised about a defendant's fitness to plead. The 1991 Act requires that a court which has determined that an individual is unfit to plead is to conduct a 'trial of the facts' to find out whether the accused committed the offence as charged. In respect of each charge not proved, the court will have to acquit the accused. The second main change is to remove the requirement that a defendant found unfit to plead or guilty by reason of insanity be admitted to a hospital. An accused found unfit to plead but also found not guilty of the offence will be acquitted. In all other cases, except where the sentence for the offence is mandatory, the court now has four options for the disposal of the person:

- to admit to hospital with or without a restriction order of limited or unlimited duration;
- to discharge absolutely;
- a Guardianship Order under Section 37 of the Mental Health Act 1983;
- a Supervision and Treatment Order requiring the accused to co-operate with supervision by a social worker, or a probation officer, for a period of not more than 2 years, and with treatment by a registered medical practitioner.

The last of these options is a useful innovation and several case examples of how this has worked in practice for the benefit of an accused have already been recorded (Dolan and Campbell, 1994; Tomison, 1992). The Order cannot be made unless the Supervising Officer is willing to undertake the supervision nor unless arrangements have actually been made for the accused to receive the treatment that is to be specified in the Order.

The insanity defence

Once a defendant puts his state of mind in issue, the decision of whether he has raised the defence of insanity is a matter of law for the judge. The conditions of defect of reason and disease of the mind are legal rather than medical concepts and have been jealously guarded as such by the courts. There are a number of cases, described below, in which little attention was given to the wisdom of modern medicine. The antagonism between the two disciplines of law and psychiatry was probably most visible in the trial of Peter Sutcliffe – the 'Yorkshire Ripper'. The psychiatrists' evidence was attacked with great zeal by the prosecution, and 'the normal courtesies were omitted until the Judge intervened' (Kay, 1993). Sutcliffe was sentenced in the normal way and was sent to prison until his illness became unmanageable and a transfer to a Special Hospital became inevitable. The tensions between legal and medical control affect the implementation of all mental health legislation (Pilgrim and Rogers, 1994).

The scope of the defence: automatism

It is acknowledged that certain organic conditions can affect the normal functioning of the brain and lead to states of 'altered' or 'clouded' consciousness. If an accused commits a crime while in such a state, he may be entitled to an outright acquittal. In contrast, a verdict of 'guilty by reason of insanity' is dealt with by the Criminal Procedures (Insanity and Unfitness to Plead) Act 1991. In *R v. Sullivan* (1983), Lord Diplock reasserted the constancy of the McNaughten Rules over the frequent changes of psychiatric opinion and terminology:

> the nomenclature adopted by the medical profession may change from time to time ... but the meaning of the expression 'disease of the mind' as the cause of a 'defect of reason' remains unchanged for the purposes of the M'Naghten Rules ... to protect society against recurrence of the dangerous conduct.

The law in this area has developed slowly and can be divided into the defences of insane automatism and non-insane automatism.

Insane automatism

In *R v. Kemp* (1956), the defendant made an irrational and motiveless attack upon his wife, severely wounding her. He offered evidence that he was suffering from arteriosclerosis that was likely to cause congestion of the blood in the brain and temporary loss of consciousness. He was found not guilty by reason of insanity after the judge ruled that the jury must consider the issue of insanity, that is, the prosecution could cross-examine about insanity, and that a disease or illness is a 'disease of the mind' for the purpose of the McNaughten Rules if it affects the mind, whether its origin is organic or inorganic. This case established that a defendant who introduces evidence of alleged automatism is regarded as putting his sanity in issue – whether or not he wishes to do so. The defendant cannot rely on a plea of automatism in order to escape the consequences of a verdict of insanity in circumstances in which insanity could be established.

In *Bratty* v. *A-G Northern Ireland* (1961), the defendant had taken off a girl's stocking and strangled her with it. There was medical evidence that he was suffering from psychomotor epilepsy, which might have prevented him knowing the nature or quality of his act. This was held to be evidence of insanity and, this being a House of Lords decision, authoritatively established the distinction between insane and non-insane automatism. The approach to be adopted is as follows:

- If the only evidence of the alleged automatism is a disease of the mind, the plea must be treated as one of insane automatism and the McNaughten Rules apply.
- If there is evidence that the automatism was due to some other cause, that is, an external factor, the plea must be treated as non-insane automatism and cannot be withdrawn from the jury.
- The judge must decide, as a matter of law, whether the plea is to be treated as one of insane or non-insane automatism.

Their Lordships made it clear that, although when the accused pleads non-insane automatism the persuasive burden of proof is firmly placed on the prosecution, such a plea will never be left to the jury until a 'proper foundation' is laid by the accused. It was stated that any:

> physical or mental illness that has manifestations of violence which are likely to recur should be termed a disease of the mind, since it is necessary that persons who are liable to uncontrollable outbursts of violence should be placed under restraint rather than obtain an unqualified acquittal.

In the case of *R* v. *Sullivan* (1983), the defendant claimed, in defence to a charge of wounding with intent to cause grievous bodily harm, that he was recovering from an epileptic fit and did not know what he was doing. However, when the judge ruled that the plea amounted to one of insanity, the defendant changed his plea to one of guilty. The Court of Appeal dismissed his appeal against the ruling. The House of Lords also dismissed the appeal and restated the distinction between pleas of non-insane and insane automatism as established in *R* v. *Bratty*. The ruling in *R* v. *Kemp* (1956) was approved, and Lord Diplock stated:

> If the effect of a disease is to impair [the mental faculties] so severely as to have either of the consequences referred to in the latter part of the Rules, it matters not whether the aetiology of the impairment is organic, as in epilepsy, or functional, or whether the impairment itself is permanent, or transient and intermittent, provided that it subsisted at the time of the commission of the act.
>
> The purpose of the ... defence of insanity ever since its origin ... has been to protect society against recurrence of the dangerous conduct.

In *R* v. *Hennessy* (1989), the Court of Appeal took an approach similar to that seen in *R* v. *Sullivan*, applying it to the case of a diabetic whose neglect to take insulin and have regular meals had induced a state of hyperglycaemia. In this state, he had stolen a car. He changed his plea to guilty when the judge ruled that his plea of automatism must be treated as one of insanity. The Court of Appeal dismissed his appeal and rejected the argument that his marital problems and depression could be categorised as external factors sufficiently potent to override the fact that he had not taken insulin, which would justify a plea of non-insane automatism going to the jury.

To prove insane automatism, the prosecution must establish that the defendant was suffering from a disease of the mind and that this induced a defect of reason. In *R* v. *Clarke* (1972), the defendant pleaded not guilty to stealing from a shop on the ground that she was absent-minded as a result of a depressive illness. The judge ruled that her pleas must be treated as insane automatism. She changed her plea to guilty and was convicted. On appeal, her conviction was quashed. The court stated that, for the purpose of the defence of insanity, by reason of a disease of the mind, she must have been deprived of her powers of reasoning; absent-mindedness did not amount to insanity. This decision satisfies the judicial guidelines for when a ruling in favour of insane automatism is required. This lady's mental state may have been prone to recur, but it had not manifested itself in an act of violence nor was it likely to do so.

Non-insane automatism

In contrast, a defendant will be acquitted where some outside force affects his state of mind, because he is not dangerous in the same way. A knock on the head, for example, is unlikely to occur again and is in effect an act of God. The evidential burden for non-insane automatism is satisfied if the defendant can show that some external factor, other than disease of the mind, might have caused the alleged automatism.

In *R* v. *T* (1989), the defendant pleaded automatism to a charge of robbery. She alleged that she had been raped 3 days previously, and medical evidence showed that she was suffering from post-traumatic stress disorder. At the time of the offence, she had entered a dissociative state with the effect that she was not acting with a conscious mind or will. The judge ruled that although there was no previous case in which rape had been held to be an external factor, such an incident could have such an appalling effect upon any woman, no matter how balanced normally, as to satisfy the requirement of a 'malfunctioning of the mind'. In addition, he ruled that a condition of post-traumatic stress is not itself a disease of the mind. The defence of non-insane automatism was allowed to go to the jury, and she was acquitted. The case of *R* v. *Rabey* (1980), in which a 'disassociative state' resulting from a 'psychological blow' amounted to insane automatism, was distinguished. It was held that the defendant's rejection by a girl with whom he was emotionally infatuated could not be treated as an external factor as the 'ordinary stresses and disappointments of life, which are the common lot of mankind, do not constitute an external cause'. The true reason for the defendant's mental condition at the time of committing the *actus reus* of the offence was his psychological or emotional make-up, which is an internal factor. Rape is an external factor and cannot be regarded as one of the ordinary stresses of life.

In *R* v. *Bingham* (1991), a diabetic had been compelled to plead guilty to a minor charge of theft because the judge had refused to allow the defence of non-insane automatism. The Court of Appeal distinguished between the condition of hyperglycaemia (as caused directly by the defendant's diabetes) and hypoglycaemia (as caused by treatment for diabetes in the form of too much insulin, or by an insufficient quantity or quality of food to counterbalance the insulin).

A plea of automatism in the form of hyperglycaemia may result in a verdict of 'not guilty by reason of insanity', but automatism in the form of hypoglycaemia must be regarded as being caused by an external factor and may result in an outright acquittal. Non-insane automatism results from something that happens to the defendant rather than from his or her physical or mental condition. This is clearly shown in *R* v. *T* (1989) as relating to psychological events and explained in *R* v. *Bingham* in relation to physical ailments. Oversensitivity to 'ordinary stresses' and events that are unpredictable and cause danger to others will not qualify for this defence.

In *R* v. *Quick* (1973), the defendant had inflicted actual bodily harm and called medical evidence to show that he was a diabetic, was suffering from hypoglycaemia and was unaware of what he was doing. The trial judge ruled that he had pleaded insanity, whereupon he changed his plea to guilty. On appeal, it was held that the alleged mental condition was caused not by his diabetes but by use of insulin prescribed by the doctor. This was an external factor, and the defence of automatism should have been left to the jury. Conversely, if his diabetes had caused the condition, the defence would have been insanity.

Proposals for reform

The ruling in the 1984 Sullivan case sparked off much criticism of the McNaughten Rules, with calls and recommendations that Parliament reconsider the question of insanity (Hamilton, 1986). There is clearly something gravely wrong when, as in Clarke, Quick and Sullivan, a person who on the evidence is not guilty will plead guilty to the charge rather than submit to the verdict of not guilty on grounds of insanity (Smith and Hogan, 1992). The rules relating to insanity clearly demonstrate the social protection role of the criminal law. Lord Diplock made this function quite clear in his judgement in Sullivan in the House of Lords:

> The purpose of the legislation relating to the defence of insanity, ever since its origin in 1880, has been to protect society against the recurrence of the dangerous conduct.

In practice, the insanity defence is rarely used (*R* v. *Bailey* (1983)). It is usually raised at the sentencing stage, severely ill offenders being advised to plead guilty to enable a psychiatric as opposed to a penal disposal.

The Butler Committee believed that the insanity defence should be retained but reformulated in order to allow psychiatrists to state the facts of the defendant's mental condition without being required to pronounce on the extent of his responsibility for the offence. The Committee proposed a new special verdict worded as 'not guilty on evidence of mental disorder', changing the words from 'by reason of insanity', which suggests a causal connection. This special verdict was to have two elements. First, the defendant could be acquitted if he were found to be mentally disordered because this would negate the *mens rea* necessary for the offence. This would apply to any mental disorders that currently came within the sphere of insane automatism. Second, the Committee proposed that, if the defendant were suffering from severe mental disorder or mental subnormality, but could not come within the first element as he or she was able to form the intent, the special verdict would apply. The Committee carefully defined severe mental disorder and subnormality on lines that equate with psychosis:

> The mental condition should be of such a severity that the causal links between the offence and the defendant's mental state could safely be presumed, and the condition should be severe enough of itself to limit criminal responsibility.

To ensure that the special verdict worked, the Committee also proposed a new discretionary power of disposal.

The above recommendations of the Butler Committee have received much criticism. It has been said that the jurisprudential basis for the proposals is weak (Wells, 1983) and that there are great difficulties created in deciding who would come within the classification of 'severe' mental disorder (Ashworth, 1975). The only practical difference that the recommendations would make is that some offenders would be admitted to hospital as technically innocent people. Under the proposals, the court would not be able to impose a prison sentence on someone found 'not guilty on evidence of mental disorder'. In a recent review of the outcomes of the Butler recommendations, Walker (1991) concluded that 'not one of its features has been adopted'. The review undertaken by the Butler Committee is still accepted as an important landmark in the development of the relationship between the criminal justice system and psychiatry, and is essential reading for students of law and psychiatry.

Diminished responsibility

In cases of murder, a new defence of diminished responsibility was introduced by the Homicide Act 1957, Section 2(1), which provides that a person should not be convicted of murder:

if he was suffering from such abnormality of mind (whether arising from a condition of arrested or retarded development of mind or any inherent causes or induced by disease or injury), as substantially impaired his mental responsibility for his acts or omissions in doing or being a party to the killing.

The defendant has to provide evidence that he was suffering as above, and if he does so, he will be convicted of manslaughter (Section 2(3)) if found guilty.

In early cases where this defence was raised, it was held that it was sufficient for the judge to leave it to the jury to decide whether the defendant's mental state was within the scope of Section 2. It now seems clear that such a ruling is wrong. In *R* v. *Byrne* (1960), the jury was directed that evidence of suffering as a sexual psychopath, caused by arrested development of the mind, which resulted in violent and perverted desires, could not amount to 'diminished responsibility'. In substituting a verdict of manslaughter for that of murder, the Court of Appeal distinguished between the cognitive and volitional aspects of the mind and for the first time allowed the condition of 'irresistible impulse' to be capable of amounting to a defence within Section 2. Lord Parker stated that:

'Abnormality of mind', which has to be contrasted with the honoured expression in the M'Naghten Rules 'defect of reason', means a state of mind so different from that of normal human beings that the reasonable man would term it abnormal. It appears to us to be wide enough to cover ... activities in all its aspects, not only the perception of physical acts and matters and the ability to form a rational judgement of whether an act is right or wrong, but also the ability to exercise will power to control physical acts in accordance with the rational judgement.

It was thought to be sufficient that the impulse experienced by the defendant gave him substantially greater difficulty in controlling it (or in this case failing to control it) than would be experienced in similar circumstances by an ordinary man not suffering from mental abnormality. The effect of the ruling in Byrne is that earlier judicial attitudes to Section 2 must now be incorrect. Subsequently, in *R* v. *Terry* (1961), the Court stated:

In the light of Byrne it seems to this Court that it would no longer be proper merely to put the Section before the jury, but that a proper explanation of the terms of the Section as interpreted in Byrne ought to be put before the jury.

In *R* v. *Seers* (1984), the defendant pleaded that a chronic reactive depressive illness could amount to an 'abnormality of mind' within Section 2. A conviction for manslaughter was substituted on the grounds of a substantial misdirection on diminished responsibility, which, following Byrne, is not to be equated with partial or border-line insanity. The Court stated that there are cases such as this in which the defendant is suffering from a condition amounting to an 'abnormality of mind' within Section 2, but which does not easily relate to any of the generally recognised types of insanity in the broad sense.

Diminished responsibility cannot be pleaded when a condition is self-induced. In *R* v. *Tandy* (1987), it was held that, with regard to the defendant's alcoholism, the defence of diminished responsibility as opposed to that of intoxication was not available if she had merely not resisted the impulse to drink. This reflects the overall judicial policy of allowing evidence of voluntary intoxication as negating *mens rea* in only a limited category of cases.

There are many problems with diminished responsibility as a defence. The terms used in the Homicide Act 1957 are very old, having their origins in disused legislation, and have been imported into the Act 'without explanation, as though two statutes will employ the self-same definition with the same clarity of effect' (Muller, 1961). Consequently, judges and psychiatrists have responded to the defini-tions in widely varying ways. Griew (1988) states that:

> Psychiatrists rather more than lawyers, have agonised over the statutory expres-sions, have looked unavailingly to the lawyers for enlightenment, and have contributed to the inconsistency in the use of the Section by the differences in their own reading of it ... There can be little doubt that the fate of some people charged with murder since 1957 has turned on the qualities of robustness and sophistication shown by those professionally involved in their cases.

However, it is also suggested by Griew (1988) that the Section 'as it stands is so badly worded that it can be made to work, and to work better than the framers intended.' In spite of all its difficulties, research shows a relatively small percentage (13%) of cases in which there was disagreement in the potentially highly contentious matters (Dell, 1984), much of the disagreement being accounted for by the fact that 'doctors routinely testify on matters not within their compe-tence'. The research also demonstrated that, in spite of increasing numbers of homicides in England and Wales from 1964 to 1979, the proportion of men who have their convictions reduced to manslaughter by reason of diminished responsibility has remained constant at 20%.

The defence of diminished responsibility has been successfully pleaded in cases where a defence of insanity would not have succeeded and has done something to compensate for a lack of 'an insanity defence that can be used' (Dell, 1983). It is surprising that the number who escape a murder conviction on grounds of their abnormality has not altered, and it has similarly been shown that the proportion of people found insane on indictment and the proportion acquitted on grounds of insanity have sharply declined. It has been suggested that the reason for this is that people who were formerly found insane on indictment or acquitted on grounds of diminished responsibility now plead diminished responsibility instead, and that only a very few people escape conviction who would not have done so before 1957.

It must be remembered that diminished responsibility is only a defence to murder and was introduced partly as a way of avoiding the mandatory death sentence at the time. The majority of the Criminal Law Revision Committee in 1979 were in favour of the retention of the defence of diminished responsibility even if the mandatory life sentence for murder was to be abolished (Criminal Law Revision Committee, 1980). This defence has worked for defendants for whom the 'insanity' defence was not available, and prior to the introduction of the 1991 Criminal Procedures (Insanity and Unfitness to Plead) Act, it was a more attractive defence as the court had a range of options to choose from when sentencing the mentally disordered offender.

Conclusions

The trial of the MDO is a much disputed and contentious area. As in all other aspects of criminal law, such debate and discussion can only serve to ensure that the best interests of justice are served. However, particular aspects of the law relating to the MDO would benefit from legislation that would bring it closer to the expertise and development of contemporary psychiatry.

The McNaughten Rules are still the cornerstone of judgements on criminal responsibility in England and Wales, and have, justly in my opinion, been the subject of critical debate as they have not changed in 150 years, reflecting the level of knowledge on mental disorder at that time. There have been many advances in medical science, in both understanding and treating mental disorder, but the strict adherence of the judiciary to the Rules makes the legal interpretation of mental disorder appear outdated and often times unjust. Reform of the present position seems to be far from the judiciary's mind, as the Sullivan case would indicate, and there has instead been a consolidation of the McNaughten Rules. The introduction of the Criminal Procedure (Insanity and Unfitness to Plead) Act 1991 has made for significant advances in the trial of the MDO as it ensures that a trial of the facts must now occur and a medical diagnosis must be heard before the jury can return a verdict of 'insanity', also introducing a flexible range of sentencing. However, without explicit reference to the reform of the McNaughten Rules, it is likely that some controversial decisions will continue to emerge from the courts.

References

Ashworth AJ (1975) The Butler Committee and criminal responsibility. Criminal Law Reports, pp 687–96.

Criminal Law Revision Committee (1980) Fourteenth Report: Offences Against the Person. Cmnd 7844. London: HMSO.

Dell S (1983) Wanted: an urgent insanity defence that can be used. Criminal Law Reports, pp 431–7.

Dell S (1984) Murder into Manslaughter. Maudesley Monograph 27. Oxford: Oxford University Press.

Department of Health (1961) Special Hospitals: Report of a Working Party (The Emery Report). London: HMSO.

Department of Health and Home Office (1992) Review of Health and Social Services for Mentally Disordered Offenders and Others Requiring Similar Services (The Reed Review). Cmnd 2088. London: HMSO.

Department of Health and Social Security (1974) Revised Report of the Working Party on Security in NHS Psychiatric Hospitals. London: DHSS.

Department of Health and Social Security and Home Office (1975) Report of the Committee on Mentally Abnormal Offenders (The Butler Report). Cmnd 6244. London: HMSO.

Dolan M, Campbell A (1994) The Criminal Procedure (Insanity and Unfitness to Plead) Act, 1991. Medicine, Science and Law 34(2): 155–60.

Griew E (1988) The future of diminished responsibility. Criminal Law Reports, pp 75–87.

Grubin DH (1991) Unfit to plead in England & Wales 1976–1986: a survey. British Journal of Psychiatry 158: 540.

Hamilton J (1986) Insanity legislation. Journal of Medical Ethics 12: 13–17.

Home Office (1964) Report of the Working Party on the Organisation of the Prison Medical Service (The Gwynne Report). London: HMSO.

Home Office (1991) Report on Prison Disturbances – April 1990 (The Woolf Report). Cmnd 1456. London: HMSO.

Kay T (1993) Voices from an Evil God. Journal of Forensic Psychiatry 4(2): 80–85 (book review).

Mackay RD (1991) The decline of disability in relation to trial. Criminal Law Reports, pp 87.

Mitchell S, Richardson PJ (1985) Archbold's Pleading Evidence and Practice in Criminal Cases, 42nd Edn. London: Sweet & Maxwell.

Mueller GO (Ed) (1961). The perception of Edwards, 'Diminished responsibility – the withering away of the concept of criminal responsibility?' in Essays in Criminal Science. Rothman..

Pilgrim D and Rogers A (1994) A Sociology of Mental Health and Illness. Open University Press.

Smith J, Hogan B (1992) Criminal Law, 6th Edn. London: Butterworths.

Tomison A (1992) McNaughten today. Journal of Forensic Psychiatry l(4): 2.

Walker N (1967) Crime and Insanity in England, Volume 1. Edinburgh: Edinburgh University Press.

Walker N (1981) Butler v the CLRC and others. Criminal Law Review, pp 595–601.

Walker N (1991) Fourteen years on. In Herbst K, Gunn J (Eds) The Mentally Disordered Offender. London: Butterworth-Heinemann/Mental Health Foundation.

Wells C (1983) Whither insanity? Criminal Law Reports, pp 787 97.

White S (1992) The Criminal Procedure (Insanity and Unfitness to Plead) Act 1991. Criminal Law Report, p 4.

Case law

Bratty v. A-G Northern Ireland [1961] 3 All ER 523, [1963] AC 386.

R v. Bailey [1983] 1 WLR 760.

R v. Bingham [1991] Criminal Law Reports 434 (JCS).

R v. Byrne [1960] 2 QB 396.

R v. Clarke [1972] 1 All ER 219.

R v. Hadfield (1800) State Tr 1281.

R v. Hennessy (1989) Times Law Reports, 31 January 1989.

R v. Kemp [1956] 3 All ER 249.

R v. Pritchard (1836) 7C & P 303.

R v. Quick [1973] QB 910.

R v. Rabey (1980) 54 CCC (2d) at 7.

R v. Seers (1984) 149 JP 124; 79 Cr App Rep 261; Crim LR 315, CA.

R v. Sullivan [1983] 3 WLR 128.

R v. T (1989) 1990 CLR 256.

R v. Tandy (1987) The Times, 23 December 1987.

R v. Terry [1961] 2 QB 314; [1961] 2 All ER 569.

R v. Young (1973) 1 All ER

Wolmington v. Director of Public Prosecutions (1935).

Chapter 11
Can medium secure units avoid becoming total institutions?

JOHN KILSHAW

The concept of the total institution, much discussed during the dein-stitutionalisation period of the past three decades, would appear to have gained a resurgence of interest as forensic mental health nursing has begun to be examined, questioned and defined – from both within and without (see, for example, Burrow, 1993; Department of Health and Social Security, 1989; Sines, 1992). It is therefore timely to review and reconsider the concept of the total institution.

Goffman defined a total institution as:

> a place of residence and work where a large number of like situated individuals, cut off from the wider society, lead an enclosed formally administered round of life.

Goffman's work on total institutions was, for the most part, informed by observations carried out during a year of field study in 1955–56 at St Elizabeth's Hospital, Washington DC, where he was employed as an assistant to the Athletics Director. Goffman's work, published in 1961 under the title *Asylums*, consisted of four papers concerning the characteristics of total institutions, the moral career of the mental patient, the underlife of public institutions, and the medical model and mental hospitalisation. In this piece of work, Goffman outlined the main characteristics of total institutions and ways of being within them.

Batch living

Most people live in a basic social arrangement in which the individual in society works, rests and plays with different people, in different places and at different times. This is in contrast to the situation within the total institution, in which each phase of the inmate's living

is carried out in the company of others, all or whom are treat[ed]
the same way. The day is organised around a strict schedule of[...]
There are formal rules and regulations that apply only to the
inmates, and there is no freedom of choice. For Goffman, batch
living is 'the key fact of total institutions'.

Binary management

Batch living facilitates a system of 'binary management' in which the
managers and the managed each have their relative positions. The
main responsibility of the managers is to ensure that the inmates
adhere to the timetable and rules and regulations. In so doing, each
group adopts a new position in which the staff members become
superior and righteous, whilst the inmates become inferior, weak and
guilty. Contact between the two groups is minimal, restricted only to
that which is necessary for the smooth functioning of the institution,
plans for inmates are kept by the staff, and little is revealed to the
inmates. Significantly, claimed Goffman, the institution is identified
by both staff and inmates as belonging to the staff, so that when talk
is of 'the interests of the institution', what is really meant is the interests of the staff.

The aim of the institution is to mould the inmate into a role that
fits the institution. This is a process of *disculturation* rather than *accultur-
ation* as the inmate is reduced from a person with the many roles of the
basic social arrangement to a person with only one role, that of the
inmate. This is accomplished through a process of 'mortification'
achieved through 'abasement, degradations, humiliations and profa-
nation of self', beginning with the admission procedures. Admission
procedures are described as 'trimming' or 'programming' because
'The new arrival allows himself to be shaped and coded into an object
that can be fed into the administrative machinery of the establishment, to be worked smoothly by routine operations' (Goffman, 1961).

Rite of passage

The new inmate is shaped and coded through an admission process
that becomes a rite of passage as he moves from one life to another.
He strips off his clothing, bathes and emerges dressed in the clothing
or uniform of the institution. He is forced to reveal his history, which
is written for others to read. As a person outside the institution, he is
able to sustain many boundaries around himself, boundaries that
protect his psyche, his person, his being, but once inside the institu-

tion these boundaries become open to abuse and violation so that 'the boundary that the individual places between his being and the environment is invaded and the embodiments of self [are] profaned'.

This happens in a number of ways. Through the practice of group or individual therapy, he may be expected to bare his soul to others. Other things (normally concealed) may be observed by others; for example, visitors may be able to see him in humiliating circumstances. If he is self-injurious or aggressive, he may be placed in a room with an observation window, into which all may peer. The inmate is never alone; he is always within earshot or eyesight of others; he may be expected to bathe or attend to his bodily elimination needs with others. Finally, he may be forced to take medication either orally or by injection.

Rewards and privileges

Within the institution there exists a system of rewards and privileges, some of which are explicit but most of which the new inmate must learn. These will be no more than the right to enjoy those things which would ordinarily be taken for granted, such as the right to possess and smoke a cigarette, take a cup of tea or coffee, or watch television. These may be small things (even insignificant everyday events outside), but in the institution they may assume much greater importance, to the extent that the day may well centre around the distribution of cigarettes. Aligned to the privilege system is a system of punishments, one set of which consists of the removal of privileges, or of the right to try to earn them. This means that privileges in the total institution are not perquisite indulgences or values but merely the absence of the deprivations one ordinarily does not expect to have to sustain. Punishments, then, co-exist with the privilege system and often mean simply the removal of privileges. The very question of release from the total institution becomes a part of the reward system. Various acts become known as ones which could mean an increase or decrease in the length of stay.

Secondary adjustment

The inmate's response to all of this Goffman describes as secondary adjustment; this can take four forms. First, he may withdraw from the situation, cutting himself off from everything except events around his immediate person. Second, there is intransigence, the inmate constantly challenging the institution by breaking the rules and refusing to co-operate. Intransigence, however, is likely to be a temporary phase, the inmate then shifting to some other form of adjustment. Third, there is colonisation: the inmate builds up a stable existence within the institution based on a limited experience of the outside world, to which life inside the institution becomes preferable. Goffman suggests that those institutions which attempt more than others to make life comfortable for the inmate must also be prepared for the possibility of colonisation. The fourth mode of adaptation is that of conversion, the inmate taking on the institution's view of himself and of what is acceptable. Some mental hospitals provided two distinct conversion possibilities: one in which the inmate adopts the psychiatric view of himself, and one in which the inmate adopts a standard of dress and a manner similar to those of the managers and assists with the management of other inmates. Conversion is the ultimate aim of the institution, at which point the inmate's personality becomes extinguished.

Goffman's approach to the study of institutions, and 'more specifically to the process by which the inmate becomes institutionalised', may be described therefore as the 'conversion approach' (Marshall-Townsend, 1971). Others who have adopted this approach include Gruenberg (1967) and Zusman (1973), the latter describing the institutionalisation process as 'social breakdown syndrome'. This syndrome, claims Zusman, has seven basic stages, the final one of which is identification with the sick. He likened this stage to Goffman's conversion adjustment:

> at some point the chronic state of sick functioning is not only accepted by the patient but he comes to see himself as like the other sick people with whom he lives and no longer looks on himself as exceptional.

Ditton (1981) noted that 'Goffman was cited by many yet examined by few.' This is certainly true in the case of his work on institutions, in which the process of institutionalisation (rather than the institution as an entity) has been focused upon. In doing so, the most common approach has been to take specific aspects of his assertions and support or contest them. Both Goffman's and Zusman's conversion theories have been challenged on the basis of studies focusing on patients' own perceptions of themselves as ill. Braginsky et al (1969) found that 78% of a sample of 189 patients agreed with the statement that most 'of the patients at a state mental hospital are not mentally ill'. From this, Braginsky concluded that, because long-stay patients did not really think of themselves as mentally ill, their decisions to remain in the hospital must be voluntary ones. On that basis, Goffman's theory is inaccurate. To avoid an oversimplification of this debate, it should be noted that Goffman stated quite clearly that inmates rarely adopted a single mode of secondary adjustment for very long; Shiloh (1971) also adopted this approach to institutionalisation, suggesting that whilst institutionalised patients had undergone a conversion, they could nevertheless accept locked wards as desirable, were more able to define a good patient than a good nurse and spoke more favourably about the hospital, stressing the recreational facilities with amenities rather than its rehabilitative practices.

Patient behaviour

In contrast to the conversion approach is a behavioural one in which explanations of institutionalisation are constructed around aspects of the patient's behaviour. One example of this is the work of Dr Russell Barton, a psychiatrist who, in the late 1950s, worked in a large London mental hospital. Barton (1959) described the condition of institutional neurosis. It is perhaps not surprising that Barton's work has had more influence and is more widely known in British psychiatry than is Goffman's. Although coming from a different ideological base, many of the themes of Goffman are echoed in Barton's work. Barton describes several factors associated with institutional neurosis, including:

- loss of contact with the outside world;
- enforced idleness;
- brutality, brow-beating and teasing;
- loss of personal contacts;
- a poor environment of care;
- loss of prospects.

Loss of contact with the outside world

The patient is locked away, often many miles from his home, and is faced with a complicated system of parole – the begrudged granting of leave often complicated by form-filling rituals. Goffman's definition contains some of these elements as his subjects were cut off from wider society and there is an inference of rules that must be learned to get leave. Visiting is often restrictive (a favour bestowed by staff) and has echoes of Goffman's assertion that the institution is owned by the staff.

Enforced idleness

Barton speaks of a lack of meaningful activity, attendants aided by one or two special patients (in Goffman's conversion approach, converted patients frequently assist the managers with the managed) who make beds and wash, shave and dress patients who are then seated at tables to be served, and often fed, a meal. The rest of the day is spent in enforced idleness until the next meal and bedtime. Much of Goffman's assertion is built around the ways in which previous behaviours are no longer possible because the institution takes them over.

Brutality, brow-beating and teasing

Barton claims that degradations lie latent in institutions. An authoritarian attitude is the rule rather than the exception and is revealed in many ways, particularly being communicated to patients in the imperative mood. Goffman also reflects on this in several ways, including the necessity for patients to beg for things, and in verbal or gestural profanities, the whole process being reminiscent of 'binary management'.

Loss of personal contacts

A loss of personal friends, possessions and personal events occurs in the mental hospital. The significance of these factors is replaced by a series of institutional possessions and institutional events. Goffman makes many references to the removal of clothes and possessions during the role-stripping process of the admission procedure. According to Barton, drugs are frequently used to control behaviour and induce apathy. Goffman refers to the use of drugs in the context of bodily contamination. The controlling use of treatment reported by Goffman is also a feature of Barton's presentation.

Poor environment of care

Barton describes the ward atmosphere, referring to drabness and the smells and noise (leading to apathy). Goffman, in relation to the contamination of bodily space, speaks of the ways in which the ward environment and atmosphere encourage withdrawal as a means of secondary adjustment.

Loss of prospects

The difficulties of a life outside the institution – finding a job, a place to live and friends – persuades patients that a life inside the institution is preferable to one outside the institution, a concept similar to Goffman's colonisation.

Deinstitutionalisation

Having defined the factors comprising institutional neurosis, the solution for Barton was simply to reverse them; he went on to expand upon how this might be achieved. Similarly, subsequent work by numerous authors (generally from a medical perspective) has focused on the process of deinstitutionalisation; for example, individualised care has been proposed as the antithesis of batch living, as Cooke (1987) advocated:

> We need a holistic, individualised care plan with which the patient is in agreement and treats the patient as a physical and emotional being.

The context of total institutions

Goffman's work drew upon reports from prisons, the services, religious retreats and other institutions but was, for the most part, informed by his experiences of St Elizabeth's Hospital, whilst Barton's work was influenced by his experience of a large, closed mental hospital. Both occurred at what could be described as the dawning of an era of enlightenment for psychiatric inpatient care. Neuroleptic medication, which relieved the more overt symptoms of mental illness, was starting to have a dramatic impact. The Royal Commission on Mental Illness and Mental Deficiency (1957) had recently reported, proposing sweeping changes to mental health legislation, in particular that persons with mental illness would be admitted to mental hospitals in the same way as general hospitals – that is, in a voluntary capacity. The point is that Goffman, Barton, Zusman and others studied and reported on a different form of psychiatric institution in a different era. Are those differences significant, and can MSUs avoid creating the total institution?

Patient empowerment

The total institution model operates from the position of separation of the two groups – the managers and the managed – the locus of power lying firmly with the managers. For Goffman, this was all important as the whole process was designed to shape the inmate into the form required by the institution. In the final decades of the century, patient empowerment is, for some, the challenge, as Ryden (1985) indicated:

> in conclusion given research findings that support a positive association between a sense of control and a sense of well being, efforts to provide a climate of self-determination seem warranted.

Implications for practice in an MSU

But can true patient empowerment ever occur in an environment in which the patient is reliant on the nurses for many services that would be taken for granted outside the institution? How many secure units do not allow patients to carry cigarette lighters, so that the patient must ask for a light for his cigarette? How many nurses need he ask before he finds someone with a lighter? And is a light for his cigarette contingent upon some form of behaviour or compliance from the patient?

Consider the simple act of having a shave before breakfast. Do patients keep their razors and blades personally? Or, before shaving, must patients ask the nurses for their razors? This process will first involve finding the right nurse, who will open a room to get to a locked cupboard containing the patient's personal razor – for which he may even have to sign.

Perhaps the ultimate expression of power lies in the control of freedom. The author, whilst in an MSU, observed the following stages involved in the simple act of going to buy a newspaper:

1. The patient asks the nurse whether he may go out 'on parole'.
2. The nurse checks the patient's eligibility for parole.
3. The nurse asks the patient where he intends to go and records the details.
4. The nurse requests the patient's bedroom key before he leaves for parole.
5. Just prior to leaving, the patient is given a parole card.
6. The nurse telephones 'control' to tell them that the patient is on the way. (If the line is engaged, the patient must wait.)
7. The nurse walks with the patient to the door to unlock it.
8. Having walked from the ward to the control area, the patient must wait for staff to open the inner of two reception doors to let him out.

9. The patient hands in his parole card to the 'control' staff and awaits their activation of the outer reception door so that he may leave for parole to buy his newspaper.

Furthermore, if the control of freedom is seen to be the ultimate expression of power, the possession of the key to that freedom may well be seen as the ultimate symbol of power. Do members of staff, consciously or unconsciously, demonstrate possession of the symbol of power by allowing a key strap to dangle, by jangling the keys in their hands or by twirling the keys on the strap like a small propeller?

How much of the patient's day is governed by time and how the institution structures time, and how many activities are carried out in the company of others because that is how the MSU operates? In other words, to what extent do MSUs function on a system of batch living? How far have we moved away from a system of binary management? MSU members of staff may have ceased to wear uniforms, but are they indistinguishable from their patients? And if the sign on the ward office door says, 'Knock before entering!', why does this only apply to patients, and how do they know this?

Do we really attempt to preserve and encourage the patient's self-determination, or is the aim one of disculturation and conversion? Do members of staff advise patients that the way to get on is to learn how to 'play the game', and how far have admission procedures moved away from those described by Goffman that lead ultimately to the process of mortification? How much do MSU staff members assist with the violation of a patient's territories? Consider the ways in which patients are required (as a prerequisite of attaining freedom) to lay open their feelings and thoughts, and to submit their secrets and bodies to treatment – sometimes without consent. Consider too the themes of rules, rewards and privileges: could it be that, if a group of patients in a MSU were asked, 'What are the rules here?', they would reply:

- 'Tidy up after yourself!'
- 'Keep your bedroom tidy!'
- 'Don't be late back from parole!'
- 'Take your medicine!'

Even where no rules are posted, most patients will have a perception of the existence of rules. How would patients within MSU services respond to the question above?

Critics of Goffman

Critics of Goffman argue that his work is one-sided and that he does not consider the reasons for the ways in which institutions behave: instead, he simply makes his observations and moves on. In addition, the changes in self-concept proposed by the conversion approach have not been empirically demonstrated. Similarly, not all total institutions portray negative characteristics, and even when mortification processes exist, they do not always have destructive implications for the self (Mouzelis, 1971). Finally, no institution is ever total in that it imports a variety of experiences of the wider external society – indeed, if it were total, it would quickly die off (Jones and Fowles, 1984).

Conclusions

Notwithstanding the critics of Goffman, and in particular the deficiencies in his methodology and sample sizes, his observations – and those of his contemporaries – should give all those in positions of power over others food for thought and provide them with a useful framework against which to examine MSU services in the age of empowerment and to avoid the excesses of the total institution.

References

Barton R (1959) Institutional Neurosis. Bristol: John Wright.

Braginsky BM, Braginsky D, Ring K (1969) Methods of Madness: The Mental Hospital as a Last Resort. London: Holt, Rinehart & Winston.

Burrow S (1993) The role conflict of the forensic nurse. Senior Nurse 13(5): 20–5.

Cooke M (1987) Part of the institution. Nursing Times 83: 24–7.

Department of Health and Social Security (1989) Report of the Hospital Advisory Service on Services Provided at Broadmoor Hospital. London: HMSO.

Ditton J (1981) The View from Goffman. London: Macmillan.

Goffman E (1961) Asylums: Essays on the Social Situation of Mental Patients and Other Inmates. London: Penguin.

Gruenberg EM (1967) Social breakdown syndrome. American Journal of Psychiatry 123: 12–20.

Jones K, Fowles AJ (1984) Ideas on Institutions. London: Routledge & Kegan Paul.

Marshall-Townsend (1971) Self concept and the institutionalization of mental patients: An overview and critique. Journal of Health and Social Behaviour, 17.

Mouzelis NP (1971) Critical note on total institutions. Sociology 5: 113–19.

Royal Commission on Mental Illness and Mental Deficiency (1957) Royal Commission on the Law Related to Mental Illness and Mental Deficiency (The Percy Report). London: HMSO.

Ryden MB (1985) Environmental support for autonomy in the institutionalised elderly. Research in Health and Nursing 8(4): 363–71.

Shiloh A (1971) Sanctuary or prison? In Wallace SE (Ed.) Total Institutions. Chicago: Aldine.

Sines D (1992) A future for Ashworth? Nursing Times 83: 36–8.

Zusman J (1973) Some explanations of the changing appearance of psychotic patients. In Price R, Denner B (Eds) The Making of a Mental Patient. London: Holt, Rinehart & Winston.

Chapter 12
Working towards patient satisfaction in forensic mental health medium secure care

PHILIP BURNARD

The field of forensic psychiatric nursing is a complex one, and there are many factors to be borne in mind when planning to ensure patient satisfaction within medium secure care. The first stage in working towards quality care must be the evaluation of the services offered to the patient. This chapter offers the findings of an evaluative study carried out at the medium secure service mental health services at the Caswell Clinic, Bridgend, Wales. The aim of the study was to explore staff views of the new unit during the first year of its existence. By exploring staff perceptions, we can begin to explore how best to ensure patient satisfaction.

The Caswell Clinic

The Caswell Clinic is an MSU that occupies a building adapted for the purpose of providing assessment, treatment, rehabilitation and aftercare for MDOs or those requiring specialist forensic services in the south of Wales. The primary task of the MSU is to provide facilities for MDOs who need care and treatment in conditions of greater security than is provided in open psychiatric hospitals. The clinic has a multidisicplinary staffing complement, inpatient and community services facilities and had 19 beds at the time of the study. The unit opened in 1992, and this evaluative study took place in 1992–93.

Method

The aim in sampling the staff of the unit was to ensure that all the staff had the opportunity to express their views. The most widely used instrument, the questionnaire, was issued to all members of the nursing staff of the MSU. This level of distribution meant that the total population of the unit, and not just a sample of the population, was surveyed.

At the beginning of the study, six staff were interviewed using a semi-structured interview schedule. Findings from those interviews were reported in the first research report. A further round of six interviews was carried out as part of the final part of the study, and findings from those interviews are offered here. The distribution of the sample for the final stage of the project is identified in Table 12.1. Confidentiality was maintained at all stages of the project, and no respondent could be identified by grade or name.

Table 12.1. Distribution of the sample for the final questionnaire survey

Grade	Frequency	Percentage
Nurse manager	1	7.1
Charge nurse/sister	2	14.3
Staff nurse	7	50
Enrolled nurse	1	7.1
Student nurse	0	0
Assistant nurse	3	21.4

Finally, 10 members of the nursing staff were invited to keep structured diaries during the 12 months of the study. The response to this diary-keeping was poor, and only four members of the nursing staff handed in completed diaries. Details from those diaries are offered in the analysis in this chapter.

Questionnaire design

The questionnaire, given to all members of the staff of the unit, comprised 24 attitudinal items to which participants were invited to respond either 'strongly agree', 'agree', 'don't know', 'disagree' or 'strongly disagree'. Room was also available on the questionnaire for participants to write their own comments. The statements in the questionnaire covered the following areas of nursing care, therapy, management and education:

• patient care;
• therapeutic activity;
• staff relationships;
• nurse–patient relationships;

- atmosphere in the unit;
- management of the unit;
- learning and personal development opportunities;
- changes in the unit.

Questionnaires were dealt with anonymously. Forty-two questionnaires were distributed during each stage of the research project. In the first two rounds, very high return rates were obtained. In the final round, only 14 usable questionnaires (33% of the total) were returned.

Diaries

Ten members of the nursing staff, of different grades, were invited to keep structured diaries. These were to be completed at the end of each month for the duration of the year of the project. Each diary contained space for the staff members' comments, under the headings outlined above, in the questionnaire section. The aim of the diary-keeping exercise was to enable staff to provide the researchers with more detailed accounts of particular happenings, or incidents that they had experienced during the year. We hoped that these would illuminate some of the consistent patterns of response found in the questionnaire findings and provide us with a more detailed understanding of the patterns of care in the MSU.

Interviews

Two rounds of interview were carried out during this research activity. In the first round, six members of different grades of nursing staff were interviewed by the researchers, who used a semi-structured interview format. The taped interviews were then content analysed, and the findings were included in the first report. In March 1993, on completion of the research period, a second round of interviews of six members of staff was carried out. These were also content analysed and the findings are offered in this report. It should be noted that it was not possible, nor was it necessarily desirable, for the same people to be interviewed in the two stages of the research.

Results

In this section, the results from all three elements of the final stage of the research project are offered. Under each heading, the findings are laid out as follows:

- responses to the questionnaire items;
- comments and summaries from the interviews and diaries.

Patient care

A range of responses to questions about patient care were elicited during the study, most of which were positive (Table 12.2). Almost without exception, staff felt that a high level of care was offered during the year of the study. They were pleased and proud to be part of the new team and often very favourably compared the standards of care in the MSU with those of the hospitals in which they had previously worked. Occasionally, it was felt that staff could not offer as much to their patients as they would have liked because of staff shortages and, for one period, because of shortages caused by maternity leave.

Table 12.2. Patient care

Choice	Score	Percentage
Patients are well cared for in the unit		
Strongly agree	10	71.4
Agree	3	21.4
Don't know	1	7.1
Disagree	0	0
Strongly disagree	0	0
Patients' needs are met by the staff in the unit		
Strongly agree	2	14.3
Agree	10	71.4
Don't know	2	14.3
Disagree	0	0
Strongly disagree	0	0
Patients exercise a reasonable degree of decision-making regarding their care		
Strongly agree	6	42.9
Agree	8	57.1
Don't know	0	0
Disagree	0	0
Strongly disagree	0	0

Viewing the situation across the year, it became clear that some views about patient care changed as the year progressed, and this was particularly reflected in the diaries that were kept. As time progressed, it became more clear that staff became more 'comfortable' in their work and involved patients more directly in their own care. Patients were encouraged to take responsibility for aspects of their care, and some staff were innovative in setting up rating scales, learning packages and support systems. All of this seems to have developed at ward level with encouragement from management. Indeed, it would seem that, from the very early days, a decision was made to encourage staff to be innovative with regard to planning patient care. It was clear that staff were afforded a considerable measure of responsibility for the activities that they developed.

A number of factors appeared to influence patient care more negatively throughout the year. At times, the level of staff was a cause for concern and resulted in some patients not being able to attend appointments at their local hospitals or not being able to use their parole appropriately. Also, at least one respondent expressed concern that, in these circumstances, 'quieter' patients were over-looked and their needs not catered for. The question of staffing levels was a recurrent one on all levels of the study and at all three data collection points.

Another respondent commented on the need to remember both physical as well as psychological care, saying that a holistic approach to health promotion and care should be encouraged:

> I feel that psychiatric nurses forget that people have a body attached to their head.

The openness of communication between staff and patients was commented on as follows:

> The patients see what is written about them and also they can write about themselves. The changeover is done with the patient [present] so that there are subjective and objective views expressed.

The recording and organisation of patient care were generally felt to be good. One respondent commented as follows:

> Care plans have been individually written for the patients (who may also sign their care plans). A key worker system has been implemented.

However, it was sometimes felt that senior clinical staff gave too much responsibility to junior staff. One of those junior staff reported as follows:

> one patient absconded. I feel that if the patient had received more support from more senior staff ... their absenteeism may have been avoided.

The organisation of the off-duty rota and of ward work occasionally came in for comment. A particularly poignant example was the following:

> male patients are not taken into account when allocating off-duty. On the day
> of the rugby international, only females were on duty.

The 'style' of patient care used in the MSU was commented on positively by a number of respondents. One discussed how crises seemed to be dealt with in an organised and controlled fashion. There was an emphasis on talking to the patient in a calm manner, and difficult situations were defused skilfully. There was a reluctance to talk about issues such as seclusion and intramuscular medication, but it became apparent that a less custodial approach was used in this unit despite the fact that it was a controlled environment.

Other comments were made about how individual patients were cared for. Each patient had his own room, which was lockable from the inside (although this could be overridden by staff in emergencies). This facility afforded the patients greater personal space and seemed to help to build up trust between staff and patients.

Therapeutic activity

The question of whether or not a forensic unit should be therapeutic as well as custodial remains a complicated and fraught one. This seemed to be reflected in some of the respondents' reports and comments (Table 12.3).

One of the most noticeable points was that the idea of 'therapy' was often construed in terms of 'patient activities' such as 'fruit-picking', 'relaxation', 'cooking' and 'walking in the grounds'. Whilst it is acknowledged that all of these things can be therapeutic and are obviously relevant to patient rehabilitation, they do not encompass the whole of what 'therapy' might involve. Little mention was made of specific types of psychotherapy or counselling, although a number of respondents pointed to the way in which particular staff members used interpersonal skills. Other respondents made reference to groups of various sorts. Examples of groups offered within the unit were:

- a leavers' group;
- a men's group;
- a women's group;
- a drug and substance abuse group.

Table 12.3. Therapeutic activity

Choice	Score	Percentage
There is a therapeutic atmosphere in the unit		
Strongly agree	0	0
Agree	11	78.6
Don't know	3	21.4
Disagree	0	0
Strongly disagree	0	0
Patients seem likely to benefit from their stay in the unit		
Strongly agree	3	21.4
Agree	11	78.6
Don't know	0	0
Disagree	0	0
Strongly disagree	0	0
Patients generally seem happy with the care they receive		
Strongly agree	1	7.1
Agree	12	85.7
Don't know	1	7.1
Disagree	0	0
Strongly disagree	0	0

Some respondents, however, felt that these groups occasionally 'lacked structure'. It might also be noted that if the group is called 'drug and substance abuse group', some consideration should be given to commissioning advice from a specialist in this field.

Some respondents noted a lack of therapeutic activity in the unit:

> There is not enough therapy work in the unit.
> There is a distinct lack of structure and therapeutic activities in what is supposed to be a rehabilitation unit.

On the other hand, another respondent commented on the level of commitment and involvement of the staff:

> The staff generally, spend large amounts of time personally on the ward without taking it back and have developed close therapeutic relationships through this contact.

On the whole, the term 'therapeutic' seemed, in the context of the MSU, to refer more to a set of personal relationships with patients than to a particular model or way of conducting therapy. Also, therapeutic activities were often of the 'recreational' and 'diversionary' sort. These have been the traditional norms and patterns of care in the psychiatric nursing field, and it might be time to consider more 'active' and 'psychological' approaches to therapy. This may be a fruitful area for further research and nursing practice development.

Staff relationships

As might be expected during the setting up of a new unit, there were times during the year when staff experienced personality clashes and differences of opinions over how the unit should be organised and run (Table 12.4). A critical and difficult period seemed to have occurred during the staff grading period. At this time, there were differences of opinion over who should have been awarded particular grades and about the ways in which the grading exercise had been carried out. This may reflect the countrywide differences of agreement about these particularly thorny issues. As a rule, staff felt positive about staff relationships – particularly at ward level. A greater divergence of views was seen at the interface of ward staff and management staff. As we shall see later in the chapter, 'management' was sometimes seen as being a little distant from ward-level staff.

In the early days of the project, there were often comments about individual members of staff, and personality differences seemed to

Table 12.4. Staff relationships

Choice	Score	Percentage
The staff in the unit work well together		
Strongly agree	3	21.4
Agree	10	71.4
Don't know	1	7.1
Disagree	0	0
Strongly disagree	0	0
Decision-making in the unit is usually multidisciplinary		
Strongly agree	1	7.1
Agree	10	71.4
Don't know	0	0
Disagree	3	21.4
Strongly disagree	0	0
I feel safe working with other staff in the unit		
Strongly agree	6	42.9
Agree	8	57.1
Don't know	0	0
Disagree	0	0
Strongly disagree	0	0

be most acute during the middle phase of the project. Towards the end of the year, it appeared that problems between staff had been worked through. However, a sense of 'us and them' between clinical staff and management seemed to persist throughout the period of the study. A small proportion of 'poor relationships' continues to exist, but staff generally appear to work well together. Reports under this heading were often very positive:

> We have become closer and more reliant on each other.
> Relationships are very good indeed.

One feature of life in the unit that was favourably commented upon was the fact that staff often met in the evenings for social events. One respondent reported that this boosted morale on occasions.

Nurse–patient relationships

There were real attempts at developing close and open relationships with patients and at encouraging patients to be involved in their own care and decision-making (Table 12.5). These factors were constant throughout the study. Indeed, a major feature of the study was the frequency with which the high quality of patient care was commented upon by all grades of staff. It sometimes seemed that problems in the unit were more frequently between staff and staff rather than staff and patients. It was clear that trust and honesty were seen as the bases for nurse–patient relationships. The emphasis on good and relatively 'equal' relationships between staff and patients was summed up by the respondent who said:

> Patients are seen as equals and apart from the obvious clues (keys etc) it is difficult to differentiate between patients and staff.

Another respondent reported that:

> Patients and staff eat, drink and cook together, share meetings and therapeutic community techniques are employed as far as possible given the secure environment.

Atmosphere in the MSU

There is a variety of indices for measuring the atmosphere of a unit, and the methods employed in this study necessarily tackle only some of the more subjective elements. 'Atmosphere' may be influenced by a number of factors, including many of those which we have already

Table 12.5. Nurse–patient relationships

Choice	Score	Percentage
Close relationships between nurses and patients are encouraged		
Strongly agree	4	28.6
Agree	10	71.4
Don't know	0	0
Disagree	0	0
Strongly disagree	0	0
There is an emphasis on therapy in the unit		
Strongly agree	1	7.1
Agree	8	57.1
Don't know	0	0
Disagree	5	35.7
Strongly disagree	0	0
I feel able to talk to other staff members about my relationships with patients		
Strongly agree	2	14.3
Agree	11	78.6
Don't know	1	7.1
Disagree	0	0
Strongly disagree	0	0

discussed: staff–patient relationships, staff–staff relationships, the organisation of the environment and so on. The atmosphere in the unit was in general described in positive terms, and most people felt that they enjoyed working in the unit (Table 12.6).

Throughout the year, the atmosphere in the unit altered. There were one or two 'crisis' points. On one occasion, a recently admitted patient died on further admission to a general hospital, and there were certain occasions on which patients absconded. There were times too when the number of acutely ill patients was high. Also, there was a period in which maternity leave seemed to be high. All of these factors appeared to affect staff morale, and the atmosphere was at times described as 'tense', 'stifling' and 'unpleasant'. Overall, however, despite these troughs, respondents' comments about the atmosphere on the unit were usually positive. It was variously described as 'relaxed', 'pleasant' and 'therapeutic'.

Management of the MSU

There were mixed feelings about aspects of management in the MSU (Table 12.7), and these were reflected in findings from all three of the data sources.

Table 12.6. Atmosphere in the medium secure unit

Choice	Score	Percentage
I generally enjoy coming to work in the unit		
Strongly agree	4	28.6
Agree	7	50
Don't know	3	21.4
Disagree	0	0
Strongly disagree	0	0
There is usually a cheerful atmosphere in the unit		
Strongly agree	1	7.1
Agree	7	50
Don't know	3	21.4
Disagree	3	21.4
Strongly disagree	0	0
I imagine that most staff feel safe in the unit		
Strongly agree	1	7.1
Agree	9	64.3
Don't know	3	21.4
Disagree	1	7.1
Strongly disagree	0	0

Table 12.7. Management of the medium secure unit

Choice	Score	Percentage
The unit is generally well managed		
Strongly agree	0	0
Agree	3	21.4
Don't know	4	28.6
Disagree	6	42.9
Strongly disagree	1	7.1
Managers seem prepared to delegate work appropriately to other staff		
Strongly agree	0	0
Agree	9	64.3
Don't know	2	14.3
Disagree	3	21.4
Strongly disagree	0	0
Managers seem to make appropriate management decisions		
Strongly agree	0	0
Agree	4	28.6
Don't know	7	50
Disagree	3	21.4
Strongly disagree	0	0

One respondent commented that the uncertainty over the future funding of the unit influenced morale. As the year progressed, however, and as the financial situation became a little more clear, so the atmosphere improved and became more positive. The same respondent also noted an essential tension between:

> a sophisticated attempt to deliver a quality service for MDOs clashing head-on with ... crude financial management.

However, other criticisms of management were noted by those who worked directly with patients. Sometimes, management seemed distant from the workplace, one respondent commenting that:

> Senior staff are critical, analytical in content and very rarely praise. This is normally given by other team members, of other disciplines.

Another suggested that:

> There is a tendency to operate a very critical, authoritarian management style.

Whilst another noted that:

> Most disharmony in the unit appears to be related to differences in management styles amongst the senior staff. There are so many 'chiefs' the poor 'indians' are often running round in circles. Better communication and an appreciation by managers of the ward level problems, stresses, etc. would lead to more effective working relationships.

However, all this should be viewed against the background of a recurrent theme – the perceived shortage of staff. Criticisms of management were often linked to these perceived staff shortages:

> Staffing levels are frequently insufficient to accommodate patient paroles.
> I feel that staff are quickly becoming disillusioned and angered by poor management and unsatisfactory staffing levels.

Notwithstanding these criticisms of the management structure, there is clear evidence that people are appreciative of those with whom they work. For example, one respondent suggested that:

> I have never worked with such a knowledgeable and motivated group of staff before.

Learning and personal development

From the beginning, there appears to have been a very positive policy with regard to personal development and education within the MSU (Table 12.8). A number of staff have registered on degree programmes, and others are booked to register in the coming year. Half way through the research period, a nurse teacher was appointed to help to develop educational policies within the unit. This appointment appeared to remotivate a number of respondents, who commented on the progressive nature of this appointment.

Table 12.8. Learning and personal development

Choice	Score	Percentage
I have been encouraged to continue my education while being employed in the unit		
Strongly agree	2	14.3
Agree	8	57.1
Don't know	1	7.1
Disagree	3	21.4
Strongly disagree	0	0
Most nurses are still developing their therapeutic skills while working in the unit		
Strongly agree	1	7.1
Agree	12	85.7
Don't know	1	7.1
Disagree	0	0
Strongly disagree	0	0
My learning needs have been discussed with senior nurses		
Strongly agree	4	28.6
Agree	10	71.4
Don't know	0	0
Disagree	0	0
Strongly disagree	0	0

A group of staff made personal efforts to facilitate their own development. A number wrote papers for publication; others contributed chapters to books and gave papers at national conferences. Generally, most respondents had positive comments to make about education within the MSU. What was particularly impressive was the range of courses on which staff were enrolled and the level of support that all levels of staff were afforded by management. Staff were enrolled on Master's degree courses, counselling courses, dramatherapy courses and a range of others.

An interesting point arises here: if there is some question of whether or not therapy is being conducted in the unit, it may be advisable to ensure that nurses are guided into taking the appropriate courses for their work as nurses. It seems vital that all courses are geared directly towards patient care, and this may mean that a more selective approach is taken towards the authorisation of course admission. On the other hand, this may also be a question of the availability of courses. It is one thing to identify a specific educational need and another to match that to a local course. One respondent offered a particularly detailed summing-up of the educational and development aspects of the unit as personally perceived:

> I feel that I am learning new things every day – skills that I have learned while training had been pushed to the back of my mind. I can now use these. I feel I am gaining confidence in my own abilities and learning new skills from my colleagues and patients. They have taught me how important it is to treat people with respect and dignity as they have not experienced this before. It made me aware of how a few kind words or normal, everyday politeness as we see in the community, can make such a difference. It does not cost anything to be polite to others.

This seems to summarise many of the best points that emerged from the study: that the unit focuses on providing a high standard of care; that nurse–patient relationships are prized; and that there is an emphasis on further education and the development of staff.

Changes in the MSU

It was inevitable that, in the first year of operation, many changes would be seen throughout the unit. There had been a policy of employing staff who had not necessarily worked in forensic settings before, and this must have meant that many staff had to go through a 'settling in' period. This is reflected in many of the comments reported in the diaries. Indeed, at least one respondent commented on the fact that keeping the diary was a useful way of monitoring and managing change.

As the year unfolded, some respondents noted that staff seemed happier to take on more responsibility. They required less direct supervision and showed considerable initiative and confidence in the setting-up of a range of groups and activities that were patient centred.

As might have been predicted, there appeared to be a 'honeymoon' period when the unit first opened that was followed by another period of some disruption and disagreement amongst staff. As they confronted new situations, and policies had to be developed, so the rules had to be written afresh. There had been no precedents for certain situations, which meant that some problem-solving strategies had to be learnt as the unit developed.

There was general disagreement with the idea that all staff were involved in the change-making process in the MSU (Table 12.9). The degree to which it is reasonable for all staff to be involved in this way may, of course, be called into question. Criticisms did, however, emerge. For example, one respondent suggested that:

> Nursing staff are not represented at policy-making groups. Senior managers have a poor grasp of staff needs.

Another respondent noted that the multidisciplinary framework that was said to be in place did not really operate and that many decisions appeared to be made unilaterally. There seemed to be a tendency amongst managers to focus on negative issues rather than to praise.

Overall, the changes that occurred during the first year of the MSU appeared to have been enjoyed by many of the staff and acted as a motivator and spur for many of the nurses. One respondent summed up this sort of feeling as follows:

> Despite the stress, this is the best place I have ever worked.

Table 12.9. Changes in the medium secure unit

Choice	Score	Percentage
Changes in policy in the unit are generally well handled by senior staff		
Strongly agree	0	0
Agree	7	50
Don't know	5	35.7
Disagree	2	14.3
Strongly disagree	0	0
Communication between different levels of staff is good		
Strongly agree	0	0
Agree	6	42.9
Don't know	2	14.3
Disagree	6	42.9
Strongly disagree	0	0
All staff are involved in the change-making process		
Strongly agree	0	0
Agree	2	14.3
Don't know	4	28.6
Disagree	8	57.1
Strongly disagree	0	0

Conclusions

From the beginning, the MSU has offered an innovative approach to the care of those who need to be looked after in a secure environment. An initial 'core' of staff was appointed to plan the philosophy and design of the unit even before structural changes to the wards were put in place. This meant that a few people had considerable influence in creating a mould and developing a philosophy within which the unit could operate. Perhaps because of this, certain core principles seemed to have emerged and been operationalised. First, there seemed to be a deliberate decision to employ staff who did not have an extensive record of forensic psychiatric nursing experience. This meant that traditional values were not necessarily brought to the new unit. On the other hand, it also meant that some staff had to learn, fairly quickly, how to operate in difficult conditions.

In the early part of the year, most staff seemed excited about the setting-up of the unit, and a training scheme was developed prior to patients being admitted to the unit. This was run by the core group of trained staff and seemed to have been warmly received by appointees. Following this, there was a 'honeymoon' period, in which there were reasonably large numbers of staff and very few patients. This pattern changed over the year as the patient population grew. A number of staff had to make considerable adaptations to the way in which they worked and the way they felt about their work. Despite all this, certain key issues remained constant and could be identified at points throughout this study.

First, it was always clear that a patient-centred philosophy was introduced into the unit and continued to operate throughout the year. Almost all of the staff on each of the three occasions on which we collected data commented on the high standard of patient care in the unit and the positive attitude towards patients that was demonstrated by all staff. Numerous staff at different levels were able to offer us detailed examples of good practice, and these have been illustrated in the three reports. Some compared the care that they found in the MSU very favourably with what they had seen in other units and/or during their training. It was as if the MSU offered many staff the chance for the first time to put into practice patient-centred principles in a secure setting. Also, the style of organising care was one that actively tried to involve the patients in their own care. There were many references to genuine, individualised care-planning. Also, many of the clinical staff were able to introduce new ways of assessing and working with patients.

A constant theme, throughout the study, and which was perceived as having a direct impact on patient care, was the question of staffing levels in the unit. In all three sections of the project, this emerged as a regular and important concern of most of the staff. While it is difficult, from the researchers' point of view, to make any judgement about the degree to which this perception accurately mirrors a mismatch between patient needs and staff resources, it remains a real concern for those who have to work with patients. It seems likely that a more qualitative study is required in order to investigate this issue in more detail. On the other hand, there are also many other variables that have to be taken into account when studying staffing levels. Throughout the study, reference was made to levels of sick leave, maternity leave, staff attending courses and other factors that would, necessarily, reduce staffing levels for certain periods.

Another important issue emerging from the study was the question of the degree to which the unit could be described as therapeutic. As we have noted, elsewhere (Morrison and Burnard, 1992), there is often a tension in forensic settings between controlling and being therapeutic. Whilst many of the respondents in this study felt that the unit was therapeutic, when they were asked to describe therapeutic activities, these tended to be couched in terms of recreational and diversional activities. Some described a range of groups that were run in the unit, but there was little explicit reference to formal psychotherapy or counselling. Often, too, it was noted that occupational therapists were employed to undertake 'therapeutic' activities, but sometimes it was also noted that those occupational therapists found their work limited and limiting. It would seem that there is a need to clarify the whole area of whether or not there is a definite therapeutic role for nurses in the unit and, if there is, what form that therapy should take. In this study, there were confusing accounts of what did and what did not constitute therapy.

A frequent theme throughout the study was the perceived tension between the nursing staff and management staff. Senior management was often described as autocratic and rather critical in its approach to working with unit staff. This was sometimes viewed as deriving from senior management staff being 'out of touch' with problems in the wards. On the other hand, there was also praise for senior management in the way it handled the aftermath of some serious incidents in the unit. These were felt to have been handled with sensitivity and supportively.

Unit staff seemed to derive much of their support from other clinical workers, and they stressed again and again that non-clinical managers did not always appreciate their point of view. Nor were policy changes in the department always felt to be made in a democratic way. There may be good reasons for this, and it may be the case that clinical staff are not always aware of the ways in which management decisions have to be made. Perhaps a more open system of management could be devised within the MSU in which both parties would be able to communicate freely with each other. On the other hand, a number of managers felt that this was already in place. That perception was not always, however, shared by clinical staff. All this needs to be tempered by the fact that, throughout the study, almost all staff also felt that there was a positive atmosphere in the unit. It would seem that the issue of management style and application is a complicated one.

Almost all respondents were positive about the degree to which the people in the unit had encouraged them to develop their own education and personal growth.

Acknowledgements

Full acknowledgement is offered to Professor Paul Morrison and Dr Ceri Phillips, who were co-researchers on this project.

Reference

Morrison P, Burnard P (1992) Aspects of Forensic Psychiatric Nursing. Aylesbury: Avebury.

Chapter 13
Five concepts for the expanded role of the forensic mental health nurse

MICHAEL McCOURT

This chapter intends to propose a number of concepts that are asserted to be evidence of the continued emerging specialist role of the forensic mental health nurse. The concepts discussed are suggested as expanded elements of the forensic nursing role, elements that distinguish the work of forensic nurses from that of psychiatric nurses in general psychiatry. Specialty status has previously been claimed as a result of situational factors such as the nature of the client group, the offending behaviour and the predominantly secure conditions in which care is delivered (Parry, 1991; Pederson, 1988) without expressly describing the nursing role in this field. Latterly, others have begun further to explore the content of this role (Beacock, 1994; Kirby and McGuire, 1995), attempting to tease out the application of mental health skills in forensic settings. A review of the contemporary literature reveals a search for concepts within nurses' roles to justify claims of specialty status. This is also true of the various roles of forensic nurses. Because of this, it is becoming possible to consider more fully how forensic nurses are developing practices in the care of MDOs in controlled environments.

The role of the forensic mental health nurse

The political context of forensic nursing developments cannot be fully explored here. However, two important points have been made in the literature. Tarbuck (1994) warns of the ramifications of the growing internal market in health care, alluding to how forensic nursing developments will arrest if nurses are unable to assert their expertise and abilities. Burrow (1993) has called for forensic nurses to provide 'highly informed, ethical, skills based practice' and to resist reductionist edict such as the 'hopeless quest for the elimination of future dangerousness'. Both points demonstrate a significant concern that forensic nursing, in the absence of a defined and valued role, will decline into an underresourced, overly custodial service. These are important considerations and reflect an urgency for forensic nurses to define, develop and defend their contribution to health care in this field. The truism of Tarbuck's assertions has been realised with the introduction of clinical effectiveness (McLarey and Duff, 1997) as a model for demonstrating service value. Despite the ending of the internal market, it is clear that the principles of clinical effectiveness and the need to demonstrate outcome values to secure resources will remain.

Historical context

In moving the discussion forward, some understanding is required of the historical context in which developments have occurred. Forensic nursing shares the same family tree as mental health nursing, which developed from 1890 with the establishment of a 'register for attendants of the insane'. In 1920, there was a formal acceptance of mental health nursing onto the general register for nurses, and since 1951, the General Nursing Council registered mental nurse (RMN) training has been recognised as the dominant training scheme in this field (Nolan, 1990).

Forensic nursing is firmly tied to these areas of mental health nursing history. However, even though mental health nursing has, since Bedlam, historically provided care in controlled environments (Tarbuck, 1994), it can be seen that forensic mental health nursing can identify its own separate history prior to, and concurrent with, these developments in mental health nursing. From the Criminal Lunatics Act of 1800, a need was identified for providing safe custody for the criminally insane, separate from that already provided for the mentally ill (Forshaw and Rollin, 1990). This led to the establishment of two blocks at Bethlem in 1816. In 1863, the blocks from Bethlem moved to the new Broadmoor Hospital, the first criminal lunatic asylum to house 'government patients', known today as MDOs (Forshaw and Rollin, 1990).

It is not unreasonable to assert that forensic mental health nursing, with its remit for caring for those who have offended or are likely to offend, has ancestry in these events. Its history, although remaining inseparable from that of mental health nursing, has a unique strand traced through the developments of Broadmoor, Rampton and Ashworth Special Hospitals – the inception of the RSU (Topping-Morris, 1992a) – to the quite extensive 'forensic circuit' (Burrow, 1993) that exists today. What is not clear, however, is at what point the psychiatric nurse who worked with the MDO acquired the label of forensic mental health nurse. It would seem that this concept is fairly recent, arising around the mid-1980s, and was possibly the result of the lift in profile of this field provided by the inception of the RSU system. Perhaps the earliest published literature to discuss the role attributes of the forensic nurse came from Canada, with Niskala (1986, 1987) and Phillips (1980, 1983). Tarbuck (1994) found Niskala's (1986) outlined competencies for forensic nurses disappointing, and Phillip's work also failed to provide significant discussion on this specialty. It is in the 1990s that there has been a moderate explosion in the UK of literature in the area of forensic nursing.

The exploration and definition of the role of the forensic mental health nurse is now beginning to emerge more clearly in the published literature. However, significant development of this specialty is likely to come from a further increase in quality research and discussion papers, and through related advances in practice and education. Both Morrison and Burnard (1992) and Tarbuck (1994) focus on the research aspect of developments as being important for progress in this field, both to lift the 'cloud of confusion' over this area, as Morrison and Burnard would have it, and to gain acceptability within the scientific community (Tarbuck, 1994). Research in nursing should study the mission and roles of nursing (Bergman, 1990), document its unique contribution to health care and generate theories of 'special relevance' to nurses (Polit and Hungler, 1989).

This should be occurring in forensic nursing, but very few published research studies address the role of the forensic nurse. This important area for research would appear to be neglected by the specialty. Instead, the studies that are published address broader issues that provide only a limited indication of any expanded role of the forensic nurse, examples being Kitchiner et al (1992b), McGleish (1992) and Lehane and Morrison (1989). Any reference to a unique or expanded function is at best implied. It would seem timely to lay further foundations for the role of the forensic nurse through greater research as the field is new (Morrison and Burnard, 1992) and the concept of the forensic mental health nurse in its infancy.

The reluctance to engage in the study of the nursing role may derive from the aforementioned cloud of confusion surrounding roles as well as the lack of a clear body of knowledge and of a systematic methodology for delivering care (Tarbuck, 1994). Whyte (1997) questions the specialty in its entirety, suggesting that the confusion is the result of there being no subspecialty known as forensic nursing and that instead 'mental health nursing is becoming increasingly forensic in nature'. Through arguing that there is no such thing as forensic nursing, Whyte more accurately demonstrates that forensic nursing has not adequately defined or asserted its role. However, despite the lack of research-based studies, there are now a number of well-reasoned and valuable pieces of literature that discuss the role of the forensic nurse; these include work by Burrow (1992; 1993); Neilson (1992) and Topping-Morris (1992a), as well as the first dedicated model for forensic nursing (Tarbuck, 1994). The work of Kirby and McGuire (1995) provides the most recent clarification of the role. Rhetoric concerning this field of nursing, said by Tarbuck to be both a science and an art, is as crucial at this stage, as is rigorous research. It is more likely that a further explication of research, rhetoric, education and practice combined, rather than just research alone, will more significantly hone this specialty.

Conceptual framework for the role

There are now concepts in the available literature that can provide a framework constituting those elements which should be the focus of the forensic nurse's expanded role.

There is no intention to dwell on how developments should proceed around these concepts; they are merely put forward as a suggestion of one potential direction for further research, rhetoric, education and practice. The five concepts for nursing the MDO are:

- risk management;
- the use of self;
- the therapeutic appreciation of control in nursing;
- nursing interventions;
- social balance in nursing.

These concepts are not presented as being exclusive and final; instead, they are presented as one impression of current thinking on the role of the forensic nurse. A discussion of these concepts will hopefully provide further clarification and stimulate interest in developing these elements of functioning, which can be viewed as evidence of an expanded and specialist role of the forensic nurse.

Risk management in nursing the MDO

Risk management refers, ostensibly, to the management of danger-ousness as proposed in Tarbuck's model, However, it should be seen as a central and proactive concept, one which engages in risk-taking for patient benefit (McGleish, 1992). Risk management should encompass the assessment and management of a wide range of dangerous behaviours in which the MDO may be at risk of engaging. The assessment of dangerousness is asserted within the literature to be a pivotal concept of the forensic nursing role (see Benson, 1992; Burrow, 1993; Kitchiner et al, 1992b; Tarbuck, 1994). Burrow (1991) describes a range of offences that may be presented, for exam-ple violence, manslaughter, sexual offences, arson and the extreme behaviours of the 'difficult to manage' patient. Tarbuck (1994) proposes an assessment of risk that forensic nurses may employ to facilitate their management of risk, although he warns that nurses must be able to reach opinions that are 'methodologically defensible and reliable in their predictability'. This is important, but nurses must also beware of employing reductionist models of dangerousness where no reliable science exists (Burrow, 1993; Tarbuck, 1994). Kirby and McGuire (1995) outline the level of expected detail that the forensic nurse should achieve with risk assessment, highlighting this as 'a distinct forensic nursing competency'.

Within risk management, there already exist certain conventions in which the forensic nurse is actively involved. One method of risk management in forensic psychiatry is the use of graduated leave systems (Burrow, 1993), and the forensic nurse has a responsibility to contribute to the decision-making process and daily management of this system. Graduated leave facilitates increased liberty for patients according to their decreasing levels of risk, with the nurse as the main support for the patient in this process either through escorting, or the daily sanctioning of, leave. Engagement in this process entails the forensic nurse making continual judgements of the potential risk posed by patients. A rising challenge for forensic nurses is how to ensure that evidence-based judgements inform their management of risk as this will contribute to improving practice (Hollin, 1997).

The concept of risk management for forensic nurses has not been explored in the literature in any great depth. A small number of papers have considered such areas as the management of violence, including the use of seclusion and control and restraint (Lehane and Morrison, 1989; Topping-Morris, 1992b), self-harming behaviours

(Aiyegbusi, 1992; Burrow, 1991), fire-setting (McGleish, 1992) and suicide (Kitchiner et al, 1992a). Important documents exist that provide excellent guidance for forensic nursing (Doyle and Hillis, 1996), but few have been published, with some notable exceptions (McLelland, 1995; Robinson et al, 1996). There need to be greater resources and specific guidance and training for forensic nurses in this extremely important area, where too often the nurse will defer to the judgement of other disciplines less familiar with the client under the care of the clinical team.

Use of self in nursing the MDO

Both Tarbuck (1994) and Burrow (1993) promote the rights of citizenship for the MDO. Burnard (1992) encourages the forensic nurse to help and be warm and genuine as part of counselling ethos with the MDO. Burrow (1993) describes how the nurse should actively pursue the patient's needs, encouraging full participation of patients in their care with the minimum restrictions. Throughout the literature, there is a clear theme of the impact that the nurses 'use of self' can have. Yet the Ashworth inquiry (Blom-Cooper, 1992) has demonstrated that the nurse can also indulge in a 'use of self' that is pejorative and contributory to the culture of denigration it describes. The forensic nurse's use of self is one of the most underdescribed aspects in the literature. It is, however, a key underpinning principle for individual forensic nurses to continue to enjoy effectiveness in role (McCourt and Whybourne, 1994).

It would seem that there is potential for a polarised nursing response to caring for the MDO, be it therapeutic or custodial in essence. This range of attitudes may emerge from an individual's regard for the therapy versus custody concept (Burrow, 1993; Tarbuck, 1994), but what they clearly demonstrate is the powerful position that nurses are in to influence the quality of care being delivered in controlled environments. Riley (1991) highlights this and focuses on the nurse's responsibility in shaping the culture of caring environments.

When considering the position that the nurse holds regarding shaping positive or negative culture, it is surprising that the literature is scant indeed in this area. Burrow (1993), Burnard (1992) and Topping-Morris (1992a) all point to the importance of a positive application of the forensic nurse to his or her role, in particular to avoid 'the machismo and those staff with controlling inclinations' (Topping-Morris, 1992a). It is not clear how this should be achieved, whether it is through the tenets of counselling (Burnard, 1992), the philosophies of citizenship and security (Tarbuck, 1994) or some other means. One key element would appear to be a need for forensic nurses to demonstrate self-awareness and reflectivity in their practice (Tarbuck, 1994). Kitchiner and Rogers (1992) have emphasised a need for nurses to voice their feelings in adapting to a forensic role. Both these factors may contribute to an increased positive use of self in delivering forensic nursing care.

Within this area, the concepts around therapeutic boundaries require further exploration; how forensic nurses perceive and develop their boundaries with the MDO is a critical component of clinically effective care. Concerns surrounding boundaries in forensic nursing have been explored by Peternelji-Taylor (1997) with her work, and the nurse's use of self more widely, demonstrating that it is as important a component in forensic nurse practice development as any other role competency requirement.

Therapeutic appreciation of control in nursing the MDO

A positive and productive use of self as described is intrinsically linked to this concept. This concept promotes the recognition, understanding and resolution of external factors of control against a patient's individual care needs. As with the therapeutic use of security (Benson, 1992; Burrow, 1993; Tarbuck, 1994), it is aimed at fostering high-quality therapeutic care within a controlled environment. The concept of control, rather than security, is introduced to encompass a wider scope of restrictive phenomena. This still includes the physical security of controlled environments such as the security fence, locked doors, controlled entrances, the design of windows and patient accommodation (Burrow, 1993), as well as the accompanying security procedures employed by secure units. It also extends to include the legal restrictions of the Mental Health Act 1993 (Burrow, 1993), the protection of the public (Burrow, 1991; Tarbuck, 1994), control and restraint and seclusion practices (Topping-Morris, 1992), graduated leave systems and, most importantly, the nurse's response to those tensions created by the nature of nursing MDOs. This is highlighted by Burrow (1993), who stated that 'control of the environment and its degree of restrictiveness can be greatly influenced by nursing staff'.

A therapeutic appreciation of control should encourage the forensic nurse's positive use of self in minimising the deficits to care threatened by control issues. This author asserts issues of control as 'illness-related risks', a recognition of the problems being needed in primary assessments. Tarbuck (1994) attaches security needs to the individual rather than to the environment or society, thereby ensuring that any considerations of control are made with equal regard for the individual's rights. Further to this, Tarbuck emphasised the clinical application of ethics, placing a significant responsibility on the nurse to act in a manner demonstrating both a beneficence and a fidelity to the patient (Tarbuck, 1992). Advocacy is asserted by Tarbuck (1994), and this may be regarded as a principle that can help to promote the individual's needs within the constraints of the public need for protection (Burrow, 1993).

A therapeutic appreciation of control may address the therapy versus custody debate. This debate asks whether it is possible to provide individualised care whilst confining patients (Burrow, 1993). Rather than constantly wrestling with this intractable problem, this described concept encourages the notion of an enhanced recognition of all the tensions created by control. Examples of best practice within this concept are increasingly evident. Collins and Robinson (1997) outline the importance of patient privacy in controlled settings; Lugg and Doolan (1997) describe the development of self-medication in a secure setting; and both Aiken (1997) and McMurran (1996) record achieving therapeutic gains in secure care. Crucially, this concept, as demonstrated in the above literature, demands the self-awareness of forensic nurses in understanding the potential of their role in influencing the degree and nature of control in care.

Nursing interventions for MDOs

Nursing interventions in forensic psychiatry are increasingly well documented, and developments within this concept are exciting and ground-breaking. Tarbuck (1994) suggests a wide range of knowledge and skills that can facilitate positive interventions in this field, including counselling, behaviour modification, the management of dangerousness and the therapeutic use of security. Burrow (1993) suggests that the forensic nurse requires a formidable knowledge base in order to deliver therapeutic interventions across the spectrum of mental disorders and offending behaviours combined. The forensic nurse must also be able to promote the rights of patients within the complexities created by the interface between the health care and judicial systems, including a greater knowledge of the court-imposed Sections of the Mental Health Act 1983 (Burrow, 1993).

What is extremely encouraging are the numerous developments in forensic nursing care interventions. However, there remain large deficits across services of available skills and intervention resources from which forensic nurses can meet the complex needs of MDOs. Benson (1992) has observed that even forensic clinical nurse specialists are underdeveloped in their role, lacking formal training in criminology and the assessment of dangerousness. Burrow (1993) talks of the 'full gamut of general mental health nursing skills' being utilised in forensic nursing, which might beg the question of whether there are any interventions that reflect an expanded role of the forensic nurse; the author believes that there are, although the essence of the skills can be found in general mental health nursing. The shift to an expanded role is in emphasis, such as the application of a behaviour modification programme to the dysfunctional sexual behaviour of a sex offender (Burrow, 1993), in that the interventions have to be modified to accommodate both the needs of the mentally disordered patient and the unique bearing that the offending behaviour places on the individual's needs.

Forensic nursing has begun to develop specialist responses that address the combined mental health, criminogenic and social needs of this particular client group. A most promising area for such developments is with cognitive behavioural therapy work within forensic settings, as undertaken by Rogers and Gronow (1997) and Guy and Hume (1998). Promoting a needs-led services is increasingly recognised (Morrison et al, 1996), and the importance of the patient's voice is enjoying higher profile as we approach the millennium. The application of an existing skills base to specific forensic need is a more common theme, forensic addictions (Thomas, 1996) and psychosocial interventions (McCann and McKeown, 1995) being two examples.

What is required within this concept is a greater analysis of need, and nursing skills required in order to promote more strategic service, practice and academic development responses to MDOs' care needs than currently exist.

Social balance in nursing the MDO

McCourt and Whybourne (1994) refer to social balance in the forensic nurse's assessment of patient care needs. This refers to imposing the least restrictions on patients whilst acknowledging a need for public safety from those individuals who may pose some danger to others. This balance is addressed well by Tarbuck's (1994) model, which, unlike previous custodial models of security, shifts security needs to a more patient-centred locus. This balance promotes a patient's rights of citizenship, unless they 'fail to act responsibly whilst exercising those rights', including the right to be cared for in 'the least secure environment appropriate'. The principles of the Reed Review (Department of Health and Home Office, 1992) are clear evidence of this at Department of Health level. Levine (1966) discusses the judicious decision-making of the nurse on behalf of the patient, and this aspect of the forensic nurse's role promotes the concept of social balance. The forensic nurse will be involved in making decisions on behalf of the patient that involve exerting some controls as previously described. Whilst accepting this, nursing integrity will only be preserved if this occurs with the positive use of self and an appreciation of the enabling and disabling aspects of controlling.

Burrow (1993) demonstrates the conflict that nurses will face within this conceptual area of functioning. The nurses' *Code of Professional Conduct* (UKCC, 1993) requires the nurse primarily to act in the best interests of the patient. It should be noted, however, that the first objective of the Special Hospitals Service Authority (1995) was to 'uphold the safety of the public'. This juxtaposition of patient care and public safety is highlighted by both Tarbuck (1994) and Burrow (1993), these being conflicts that impinge on both the forensic nurse's professional and moral responsibilities. Tarbuck's (1994) shift of security needs to patient safety requirements (in the broadest sense) aids this balance, so that security is no longer service or public in emphasis but is expressed as part of the individual's care needs. This individual focus should militate against custodial practices and blanket policies (Tarbuck, 1994). Kirby and McGuire (1995) help the understanding of this concept greatly by ascribing a competency to address this and issues of control. It is the forensic nurses' responsibility to consider the tensions of this principle and to reflect on their practice and service delivery in order to evaluate their care against such competences.

Stage of development

Burrow (1993) asserts that it is the emphasis on offence behaviour that forms the exclusive focus of the forensic health care model. Tarbuck (1994) extends this discussion when he says, 'Two characteristics immediately set the forensic nurse apart from others ..., the maintenance of security and ... assessing and caring for the dangerous individual.' Within the tensions that these phenomena create, nurses must have an enhanced awareness of their impact on the patient care experience, with an emphasis on appreciating the concepts of control and risk management. The forensic nurse will need a formidable knowledge base and skills expertise in order to achieve the delivery of high-quality care. The forensic nurse must strive to achieve a balance of care that ensures high-quality, ethical and patient-centred care whilst placing the minimal compromise possible on public safety needs.

It is difficult to judge just how developed this specialty of forensic mental health nursing actually is. Whether it is an emerging specialty (Tarbuck, 1994) or an existing one (Burrow, 1993) remains unclear. What is overwhelming is the strength of consensus in the literature that there is evidence of an expanded role, which is beginning to provide firm foundations for the development of this specialty. There is an increasing wealth of formal training in the education or skills required for this suggested expanded role (Burrow, 1993). However, it can still be contested that existing training has yet to meet the specific needs described for achieving competency within the expanded role.

Conclusions

With limited consistency or consensus on the outline of the role and the associated practice development and training required, forensic nurses provide care within the existent conceptual tensions. More exploration of rhetoric, research, education and practice is required. Forensic mental health nurses need to define, develop and defend their roles in the care of MDOs and in effectively contributing to the policy and strategy components of this sphere of health care. At the close of the millennium, NHS changes and reforms will demand even more role clarity, and forensic mental health nurses must engage in developments that bring greater definition to their roles.

References

Aiken F (1997) Group psychotherapy in a forensic setting. Psychiatric Care 4.

Aiyegbusi A (1992) Self harm in secure environments. In Morrison P, Burnard P (Eds) Aspects of Forensic Psychiatric Nursing. Aldershot: Avesbury.

Beacock C (1994) Development strategy for forensic nursing. In Thompson T, Mathias T (Eds) Lyttle's Mental Health and Mental Disorder, 2nd Edn. London: Churchill Livingstone.

Benson R (1992) The clinical nurse specialist in forensic settings. In Morrison P, Burnard P (Eds) Aspects of Forensic Psychiatric Nursing. Aldershot: Avesbury.

Bergman R (1990) Nursing Research for Nursing Practice. London: Chapman & Hall.

Blom-Cooper L (1992) Report of the Committee of Inquiry into Complaints about Ashworth Hospital, Volume 1. London: HMSO.

Burnard P (1992) The expanded role of the forensic psychiatric nurse. In Morrison P, Burnard P (Eds) Aspects of Forensic Psychiatric Nursing. Aldershot: Avesbury.

Burrow S (1991) The special hospital nurse and the therapeutic dilemma of custody. Journal of Advances in Health and Nursing Care 1(3): 21–38.

Burrow S (1992) The deliberate self harming behaviour of patients within a British Special Hospital. Journal of Advanced Nursing 17(2): 138–48.

Burrow S (1993) The treatment of security needs of Special Hospital patients: a nursing perspective. Journal of Advanced Nursing 18(8): 1267–78.

Collins M, Robinson D (1997) Studying patient choice and privacy in a forensic setting. Psychiatric Care 4: 12–15.

Department of Health and Home Office (1992) Reivew of Health and Social Services for Mentally Disordered Offenders and Others Requiring Similar Services (The Reed Review). Cmnd 2088. London: HMSO.

Doyle M, Hillis G (1996) Risk Assessment – Guidance for Mental Health Nurses. Unpublished document. London: RCN.

Forshaw D, Rollin H (1990) The history of forensic psychiatry in England. In Bluglass R, Bowden P (Eds) Principles and Practices of Forensic Psychiatry. London: Churchill Livingstone.

Guy S, Hume A (1998) A CBT strategy for offenders with a personality disorder, Part 1. Mental Health Practice 2(4).

Hollin C (1997) Assessing and managing forensic risk. Psychiatric Care 4(5): 212–15.

Kirby P, McGuire N (1995) Forensic psychiatric nursing. In Stuart GW, Sundeen SJ (Eds) Principles and Practices of Psychiatric Nursing. St Louis: CV Mosby.

Kitchiner N, Rogers P (1992) Evaluating the preparation of forensic psychiatric nurses. In Morrison P, Burnard P (Eds) Aspects of Forensic Psychiatric Nursing. Aldershot: Avesbury.

Kitchiner N, Riach G, Robinson A (1992a) Suicide risk in three controlled environments. In Morrison P, Burnard P (Eds) Aspects of Forensic Psychiatric Nursing. Aldershot: Avesbury.

Kitchiner N, Topping-Morris B, Wright I, Burnard P, Morrison P (1992b) The role of the forensic psychiatric nurse (short report). Nursing Times 88(8): 56.

Lehane M, Morrison P (1989) Secluding patients in forensic care. Nursing Times 85(49): 55.

Levine ME (1966) Adaptation and assessment. American Journal of Nursing 66(1): 2450–3.

Lugg S, Doolan B (1997) Self-medication within a high security hospital. Psychiatric Care 4(5): 225–8.

McCann G, McKeown M (1995) Applying psychosocial interventions: Thorn initiative in forensic settings. Psychiatric Care 2(4): 133–6.

McCourt M, Whybourne L (1994) Role of the Forensic Nurse – a Discussion Paper. Unpublished document. London: Special Hospital Services Authority.

McGleish A (1992) Nursing management of fire risk in controlled environments. In Morrison P, Burnard P (Eds) Aspects of Forensic Psychiatric Nursing. Aldershot: Avesbury.

McLarey M, Duff L (1997) Clinical effectiveness. Nursing Standard 11(52): 33–7.

McLelland N (1995) The assessment of dangerousness. Psychiatric Care 2(1): 117–19.

McMurran M (1996) Managing clinical risk through treatment. Psychiatric Care 3(2):

51–5.

Morrison P, Burnard P (Eds) (1992) Aspects of Forensic Psychiatric Nursing. Aldershot: Avesbury.

Morrison P, Burnard P, Phillips C (1996) Patient satisfaction in a forensic unit. Journal of Mental Health 5(4): 369–77.

Neilson P (1992) A secure philosophy. Nursing Times 88(8).

Niskala H (1986) Competencies and skills required by nurses working in forensic areas. Western Journal of Nursing Research 8(4): 400–13.

Niskala H (1987) Conflicting convictions – nurses in forensic settings. Canadian Journal of Psychiatric Nursing 28(2): 10–14.

Nolan P (1990) Psychiatric nursing: the first 100 years. Senior Nurse 10(10): 20–3.

Parry J (1991) Community care for mentally disordered offenders. Nursing Standard 5(23): 29–33.

Pederson P (1988) The role of the community psychiatric nurse in forensic psychiatry. Community Psychiatric Nurses Journal (Jun): 12–17.

Peternelji-Taylor CA (1997) Forensic psychiatric nursing. In Johnson BS (Ed.) Psychiatric Mental Health Nursing. Philadelphia: JB Lippincott.

Phillips MS (1980) Forensic psychiatric program for nurses. Dimensions in Health Service (May): 29–30.

Phillips MS (1983) Forensic psychiatry – nurses attitudes revealed. Dimensions in Health Service 60(9): 41–3.

Polit DF, Hungler BP (1989) Essentials of Nursing Research. London: JB Lippincott.

Riley M (1991) A collective responsibility. Nursing Standard 5(33): 18–20.

Robinson D, Reed V, Lange A (1996) Developing risk assessment scales in forensic psychiatric care. Psychiatric Care 3(4): 146–51.

Rogers P, Gronow T (1997) Anger management: turn down the heat. Nursing Times 93(3).

Special Hospitals Service Authority (1995) SHSA Review. London: SHSA.

Tarbuck P (1992) Ethical standards and human rights. Nursing Standard 7(6): 27–30.

Tarbuck P (1994) The therapeutic use of security: a model for forensic nursing. In Thompson P, Mathias P (Eds) Lyttle's Mental Health and Mental Disorder, 2nd Edn. London: Churchill Livingstone.

Thomas O (1996) Substance Misuse by Mentally Disordered Offenders – Dilemma for Nurses. Unpublished document. Retford: Rampton Hospital.

Topping-Morris B (1992a) An historical and personal view of forensic nursing services. In Morrison P, Burnard P (Eds) Aspects of Forensic Psychiatric Nursing. Aldershot: Avesbury.

Topping-Morris B (1992b) A view of seclusion in psychiatric nursing. In Morrison P, Burnard P (Eds) Aspects of Forensic Psychiatric Nursing. Aldershot: Avesbury.

UKCC (United Kingdom Central Council for Nursing, Midwifery and Health Visiting) (1993) Code of Professional Conduct, 3rd Edn. London: UKCC.

Whyte L (1997) Forensic nursing: a review of concepts and definitions. Nursing Standard 11(23): 46–7.

Chapter 14
The attitudes of forensic mental health nurses

CHRIS CHALONER and CONNOR KINSELLA

> The evils arising from the generally indifferent character of attendants, and from the deficiency as to the resources they ought to possess, are so great that few things would benefit the insane more than devising some remedy for them. (Connolly, 1847)

For mental health nurses, delivering care to disturbed and potentially dangerous patients has traditionally carried a number of negative attributions. Whilst little in the way of documentary evidence exists, there remains a myth suggesting that such a role is practised by individuals whose principal orientation is towards custody rather than therapy (Kinsella and Chaloner, 1995). A number of highly publicised incidents and formal inquiries have fuelled the debate regarding the attitudes of nurses working with offender patients, particularly those within secure clinical environments (Department of Health, 1992; Special Hospitals Service Authority, 1993).

Whilst the existence of potentially negative attitudes amongst forensic mental health nurses receives frequent exposure (particularly via the tabloid press), it has, until comparatively recently, been far less common to read material that reflects the positive, therapeutic attitudes displayed by nurses working within what are (potentially) the most stressful and hazardous of clinical environments. The persistent criticisms of forensic mental health nursing must inevitably affect (either positively or negatively) the attitudes of practitioners towards their role.

It is the purpose of this chapter to present an overview of attitudes in forensic mental health nursing. Attitudes will be examined in relation to both the history of this specialty and the current climate of clinical and strategic development.

History and attitudes

The mental institutions of the eighteenth and early nineteenth centuries employed 'keepers' to attend to the needs of the mentally ill:

> The term implied that those who looked after the mentally ill both restricted access to them and controlled the movements of patients in the same way that zoo-keepers and game-keepers controlled animals and game. (Nolan, 1993)

From the mid-nineteenth century onwards, 'attendant' became the preferred terminology, possibly a semantic ploy designed to reflect a more caring role on the part of those recruited to work with the mentally ill. During an era that did not have recourse to effective psychotropic drugs, a principal concern of attendants was to control any violent behaviour exhibited by their charges. Those employed to carry out such a thankless task were, for the most part, poorly educated men and women from the lower echelons of the social class system, and the demonstration of a positive attitude towards 'care' was, perhaps, deemed unnecessary. 'Superintendents tended to look for attributes such as size or strength in potential attendants rather than for any signs of ability to relate to patients' (Nolan, 1993). The following offers some indication of how such attendants were viewed by their employers (the Medical Superintendents):

> Although an office of some importance and great responsibility, [the role of the attendant] is held as degrading and odious employment, and seldom accepted but by idle and disorderly persons. (Haslam, 1809)

Dr Haslam even goes as far as to suggest that his employees were often ineffective in the management of violent behaviour because of a tendency to 'indulge in a diet and beverage, which induce corpulence and difficulty of breathing!' Whilst it is interesting to consider the role and nature of our predecessors who were charged with the task of caring for (or managing) the mentally ill, we might suggest that any negative attitudes they maintained towards their work must surely, to some degree, have reflected the custodial and authoritarian image attributed to their prescribed role.

Despite some therapeutic and legislative reforms (including the recognition of a Mental Nurse qualification by the General Nursing Council in 1923), the care of the mentally ill, until comparatively recent times, remained focused upon the large institutions. Psychiatric nursing maintained a somewhat inferior professional standing and was regarded as an undertaking with limited professional or public commendation, associated mainly with custodial duties and tasks. There are undoubted similarities between the unfortunate origins of the attendant role and its subsequent development into that of the 'psychiatric nurse', and the perceptions that have persisted regarding those nurses who work with mentally disordered offenders (MDOs) within locked institutions.

Current situation

A traditional view of nursing practice within secure environments was that nursing care and custodial duties were mutually constitutive. An essential regard for security plus the fusion of such considerations with clinical practice assisted in promoting a perception of forensic mental health nursing as somehow less therapeutically orientated than other forms of nursing practice. Burrow (1991), referring to 'the dilemma of therapeutic custody', drew attention to the potential contradictions faced by nurses when attempting to provide therapy within the opposing conditions of client-orientated care and public protection. Forensic mental health nursing has frequently been the focus of disagreeable media attention, and newspaper reports describing high-security hospitals as 'prisons', and nursing staff as 'warders', are not uncommon. Of course, being the recipient of negative commentary is not the exclusive concern of nursing alone. Criticism is often expressed towards various professional groups concerned with the care of MDOs. These negative images have been extended by the seemingly abundant official inquiries into the care of patients and conduct of mental health services within secure hospitals and beyond (see, for example, Department of Health and Home Office, 1992; Ritchie et al, 1994).

It is conceivable that the recurrent negative commentary on the role of forensic mental health nurses and their practice may have contributed to the development of defensive attitudes amongst practitioners. In addition, the traditionally isolated physical and professional nature of forensic mental health practice may have contributed to the development of both defensive and élitist attitudes amongst carers. Until comparatively recently, forensic mental health nursing was practised within areas that were generally inaccessible to the public and indeed to the majority of health care professionals. We would suggest that a recurrent negativity concerning their professional roles must inevitably affect forensic nurses' self-perceptions.

Of course, it is a worrying, but perhaps realistic, consideration that the more negative images of the forensic nursing role may have proved attractive to certain individuals seeking an opportunity to exert power and authority in a secure and covert environment without a requirement to promote or maintain any pretence towards caring or therapeutic outcomes. In what may be regarded as a prime example of the 'vicious circle' concept, the unintentional recruitment of such individuals may have assisted in further distancing the perceived ethos of forensic mental health nursing from the majority of care settings.

It would obviously be inappropriate to excuse anything less than the highest standard of integrity amongst forensic mental health nurses. Nonetheless, it may be helpful, when considering the existence of negative attitudes amongst forensic mental health nurses, to consider the disparity between the realities of their traditional clinical practice environments and those of their more 'mainstream' colleagues. We are aware of various defences employed by nurses to protect themselves from the stress of patient contact (Handy, 1991; Menzies, 1960), and it is possible that attitudes not solely client centred and 'therapeutic' may have been socially constructed as a defence against the varied stresses of delivering care to individuals who may have committed grievous offences, and against the daily contact with the extremes of antisocial behaviour.

The many constructive developments, both practical and philosophical, that followed reports such as those of the Royal Commission (1957), the Butler Committee (Department of Health and Social Security, 1974) and more recently the Reed Committee (Department of Health and Home Office, 1992) have undoubtedly assisted in developing a more positive profile for forensic mental health nursing and in focusing attention on the more positive aspects of care within secure environments.

Attitudes and nursing

What are 'good' attitudes on the part of the nurse, and are such attitudes generally possessed by forensic mental health nurses? How might we go about measuring attitudes in nursing? First, we must determine what kinds of attitude we wish to measure.

The ENB stated, in its syllabus for registered mental nurse training (ENB, 1982), that the development of desirable attitudes is an aim of nurse training. Rolfe (1990) states that 'Clearly the desirable attitudes referred to by the ENB are attitudes held by the nurse about psychiatric illness, and in particular, towards patients'. However, the 1982 syllabus was distinctly uninformative in telling us exactly what such desirable attitudes might be. Rolfe's study attempted to define desirable attitudes in psychiatric nursing and proposed a theoretical framework for constructing an instrument for attitude measurement. He took as his frame of reference the three core principles of Rogerian psychotherapy: genuineness, respect and empathy (Rogers, 1951).

Rolfe's study attempted to pilot a test instrument based on Rogers' three principles. The instrument was applied to three small samples of nurses: registered general nurse students on psychiatric placement, second-year registered mental nurse students and trained psychiatric nurses. The results obtained were somewhat unexpected. The registered mental nurse students exhibited the lowest tendency to employ empathy, genuineness and respect, whilst the highest scores came from the registered general nurse students on mental health placements.

Other researchers have studied attitudes of mental health nurses along a 'management-centred practice – client-centred practice' continuum, in which management-centred practice is concerned with block treatments that meet the needs of the institution and the nurse rather than those of the client (Garety, 1981). It is suggested that the latter represents a situation analogous with most large institutions, but that more client-centred, individualised practice should be the norm as mental health care moves into the community.

A study of nurses completing the Management Practices Questionnaire (Conning and Rowland, 1992) showed how, when nurses were asked to assess a patient presented in a hypothetical clinical scenario, such assessments appeared to be heavily orientated towards 'management practices', leading the authors to conclude that:

> the reality may be that care is being individualised in the sense that it is unique to the staff member who makes the decision rather than being based solely upon information about the individual patient.

Probably the most widely used measure of attitudes amongst mental health nurses, and to date the only instrument to have been used to determine the attitudes of nurses working within forensic mental health environments (Kinsella and Chaloner, 1995; Squier, 1993), is the Claybury Selection Battery (Caine et al, 1982).

The Attitude to Treatment Questionnaire (ATQ) measures the attitudes of mental health nurses along a continuum ranging from a conservative 'medical model' orientation to a more liberal, socially orientated treatment outlook. The Direction of Interest Questionnaire (DIQ) distinguishes between an 'inward' or 'outward' orientation on the part of respondents. An inward orientation represents an interest in more 'psychological' matters, the arts and working with people. An outward orientation represents a tendency for an interest in more practical, objective activities and an interest in working with objects rather than people. As one might suspect, there is a strong tendency for individuals scoring high on liberalism on the ATQ to show a markedly inward-looking orientation on the DIQ. A number of studies have demonstrated the ability of these questionnaires to distinguish between attitudes of, for example, nurses working in traditional hospital settings and those working within therapeutic communities (Caine et al, 1981), and between registered general and registered mental nurse students (Clarke, 1991).

We know from previous studies that nurses working in large, older-style institutions tend towards a significantly more 'conservative' and 'biological' orientation than nurses working in therapeutic communities or in community care. Likewise, the DIQ scores of various groups suggest that more outward, 'object-orientated' nurses tend to work within the more traditional, institutional environments, whilst inward, 'psychologically orientated' nurses tend to work in therapeutic communities, etc. It is also important to note some of the correlations between attitude scales such as the ATQ and certain demographic variables such as education and age. People (of all disciplines) with a higher level of education tend to be more liberal in their attitudes towards treatment than those with fewer qualifications, hence a significant positive correlation between trained nurses and more liberal attitudes. Likewise older nurses tend to be much more conservative in their attitudes than their younger colleagues.

Squier (1993) employed the Claybury Selection Battery to investigate the relationship between ATQ and DIQ scores, 'ward atmosphere' and the behaviour of patients. The sample group were nurses working in a regional secure unit (RSU), intensive care unit and acute admission wards. Squier found no significant differences between any of the units in their ATQ and DIQ scores, although the RSU sample appeared to be somewhat less conservative and more inwardly orientated than the majority of their colleagues in other areas. In another study, the authors attempted to examine the commonly held myth that medium secure units (MSUs) are staffed by nurses more orientated toward custody than therapy (Kinsella and Chaloner, 1995). The ATQ, DIQ and a questionnaire detailing a variety of demographic variables (such as age, length of experience and educational attainments) were administered to samples of nurses working in three supposedly disparate nursing environments: MSUs, acute admission wards and drug dependence units. The research hypothesis would predict that RSU nurses were significantly more disposed toward a conservative, medical model approach, and more outwardly orientated than their colleagues in less-controlled environments.

In fact, no significant differences were found between the three groups of nurses, although individual units varied considerably from one another on the measures used, which could not be accounted for by differentials such as age and education. Whilst we can infer little from these studies, which of course have nothing to say about the attitudes of nurses in high-security forensic mental health establishments, there would appear to be little evidence so far that nurses working with offender patients show any greater tendency toward custodialism than other mental health nurses.

MSU forensic nurses

Forensic mental health nursing has never enjoyed the positive image commonly ascribed to the majority of other areas of nursing practice. It is unlikely that such practitioners would be referred to as 'angels' within the popular press; indeed, their practice appears to be highlighted only at times of controversy and public concern. This is perhaps perpetuated by the commonly held public and (non-forensic) professional view that forensic mental health nurses persist in emphasising custodial practices above the more positive aspects of therapeutic outcomes, 'success' being measured by the maintenance of security and safety rather than by therapeutic outcomes.

Whilst there remains some ambiguity regarding what constitutes good, positive attitudes in forensic mental health nursing, there would appear to be a consensus that nurses should be striving toward an individualised, client-centred and egalitarian approach. Are nurses working with offender patients able to say that they possess such enlightened attitudes? The answer is that we cannot as yet be sure. Whilst we have referred to the evidence that MSU nurses are no more 'medical model' oriented than nurses elsewhere, specific data regarding, for example, client-centredness in forensic mental health nursing has yet to be elicited.

High-security forensic nurses

Throughout this overview, we have referred to forensic nursing in quite broad, generic terms. Is this fair? The high-security hospitals in England (Ashworth, Broadmoor and Rampton) are large, somewhat isolated institutions that, over a long period of time, have developed a distinctive culture and identity. In contrast, MSUs are smaller, less physically and professionally isolated, and have developed within the comparatively recent past. It is possible that MSUs have yet to develop a discrete culture that intrinsically affects the attitudes of those who work therein.

Further areas for exploration

We have observed that there appears to be little to differentiate MSU nurses from other mental health nurses, but it would be very hazardous to attempt to generalise these results too widely. High-security nursing has been criticised for being custodially orientated, but we do not as yet have the research evidence to speculate any further on the attitudes of such nurses. This is certainly an area to be developed in order that we can ascertain whether nurses working within these environments do indeed develop 'untherapeutic' attitudes. It is to be expected that an individual's attitude towards his or her professional role will be based on a number of significant factors, for example personal and professional experiences, and individual and institutional philosophy. Of course, attitudes towards offences and offending behaviour must also influence attitudes towards practice. However, we believe that the gathering of information that assists in the identification of how forensic mental health nurses perceive their role, purpose and patients/clients can contribute to the positive development that this specialty is currently demonstrating.

Conclusions

We have perhaps raised more questions than we have answered. Within the confines of this brief overview, we have been unable fully to address all aspects of the forensic mental health role and have therefore deliberately confined our discussions to the attitudes of those who work within secure environments.

The professional scope of forensic mental health nursing is ever widening, and the attitudes of its practitioners towards their practice is a vital aspect of ensuring that both care and management practices are delivered in a manner that ensures the achievement of the established aims of the specialty.

References

Burrow S (1991) The special hospital nurse and the dilemma of therapeutic custody. Journal of Advances in Nursing and Health Care 1(3): 21–38.

Caine TM, Smail DJ, Wijesinghe OBA, Winter DA (1981) Personal Styles in Neurosis: Implications for Small Group Psychotherapy and Behaviour Therapy. London: Routledge & Kegan Paul.

Caine TM, Smail DJ, Wijesinghe OBA, Winter DA (1982) The Claybury Selection Manual. Windsor: NFER–Nelson.

Clarke L (1991) Attitudes and interests of students and applicants from two branches of the British nursing profession. Journal of Advanced Nursing 16: 213–23.

Conning AM, Rowland A (1992) Staff attitudes and the provision of individualised care: what determines what we do for people with long-term psychiatric disabilities? Journal of Mental Health 1: 71–80.

Connolly J (1847) The Construction and Government of Lunatic Asylums. London: Dawsons.

Department of Health (1992) Report of the Committee of Inquiry into Complaints about Ashworth Hospital, Volume I. London: HMSO.

Department of Health and Social Security and Home Office (1974) Report of the Committee on Mentally Abnormal Offenders (The Butler Report). Cmnd 6244. London: HMSO.(1992) Report of the Committee of Inquiry into Complaints about Ashworth Hospital, Volume I. London: HMSO.

Department of Health and Home Office (1992) Review of Health and Social Services for Mentally Disordered Offenders and Others Requiring Similar Services: Final Summary Report (The Reed Review). London: HMSO.

ENB (English National Board for Nursing, Midwifery and Health Visiting) (1982) Syllabus of Training Professional Register – Part 3. London: ENB.

Garety PA (1981) Staff Attitudes, Organisational Structure and the Quality of Care of Long-stay Psychiatric Patients. Unpublished MPhil thesis, University of London.

Handy JA (1991) The social context of occupational stress in a caring profession. Social Science and Medicine 32(7): 819–30.

Haslam J (1809) Observations on Madness and Melancholy. London: Callow.

Kinsella C, Chaloner C (1995) Attitude to treatment and direction of interest of forensic mental health nurses: a comparison with nurses working in other specialities. Journal of Psychiatric and Mental Health Nursing 2(6): 351–7.

Menzies I (1960) A case study in the functioning of social systems as a defence against anxiety. Human Relations 13(2).

Nolan P (1993) A History of Mental Health Nursing. London: Chapman & Hall.

Ritchie JH, Dick D, Lingham R (1994) The Report of the Inquiry into the Care and Treatment of Christopher Clunis. London: HMSO.

Rogers C (1951) Client Centred Therapy. Boston: Houghton Mifflin.

Rolfe G (1990) The assessment of therapeutic attitudes in the psychiatric setting. Journal of Advanced Nursing 15: 564–70.

Royal Commission (1957) Royal Commission on the Law Relating to Mental Illness and Mental Deficiency 1954–1957. London: HMSO.

Special Hospitals Service Authority (1993) 'Big, Black and Dangerous?' Report of the Committee of Inquiry into the Death in Broadmoor Hospital of Orville Blackwood and a Review of the Deaths of Two Other Afro-Caribbean Patients. London: SHSA.

Squier RW (1993) The Relationship Between Ward Atmosphere, Staff Attitudes and Patient Behaviour. Unpublished document.

Chapter 15
Clinical supervision for forensic mental health nurses: the experience of one medium secure unit

PAUL ROGERS, KEVIN GOURNAY and
BARRY TOPPING-MORRIS

Clinical supervision for nurses has become an integral aspect of health care delivery in today's health care service. Key documents are demanding that nursing services incorporate clinical supervision as a norm in practice development (Department of Health, 1994; NHS Management Executive, 1993; UKCC, 1994).

Mental health nursing has received considerable attention in relation to the need for clinical supervision. *Working in Partnership: Report of the Review of Mental Health Nursing* (Department of Health, 1994) recommended that clinical supervision be established as an integral part of practice, whilst in Wales, the Welsh Office (1996) produced *Caring for the Future: The Nursing Agenda for Mental Health Nursing Action Plan*. This identified that all mental health nursing services in Wales should have a clinical supervision structure in place by June 1997.

Furthermore, the *Report of the Confidential Inquiry into Homicides and Suicides by Mentally Ill People* (Royal College of Psychiatrists, 1996) identified clinical supervision as a requirement when providing services for MDOs. This report concluded that services need to facilitate continued professional development for all staff and recommended that services should address the extent and quality of direct staff–patient contact.

Over the past 5 years, the Caswell Clinic has been gradually developing a system for clinical supervision. This process has already been reported by Rogers and Topping-Morris (1997). This chapter provides a follow-up of this initiative and evaluates the effect of this development to date via the first annual audit of identified and agreed standards, and the survey of nursing satisfaction levels of all nurses who receive clinical supervision. A discussion of the findings is provided, as is a consideration of areas for future research and development.

Clinical supervison

Clinical supervision for nurses is an issue to which most professional organisations and Trusts have attached great importance. Trusts across the country are implementing supervision into practice, and scarcely a week goes by when it is not mentioned in the nursing press. Despite this, however, there is an absence of any well-controlled systematic studies of effectiveness. A review of the literature on clinical supervision for nurses using the database CINAHL (1983–97) identified 71 articles on nursing and clinical supervision. A crude analysis of these articles suggests that five themes exist: descriptions of particular models; clinical supervision for specific groups (for example CPNs); discussions and reviews; the experiences and perceptions of nurses; and the reduction of stress/burn-out. The lack of an empirical basis is evident throughout the literature, discussion and description being the mainstay. The research that does exist is based on models of supervision that are difficult to define, and no one has yet attempted to identify which components of clinical supervision might actually make a difference to patient outcomes.

Butterworth et al (1997) conducted a large 18-month evaluative study of clinical supervision and mentorship in England and Scotland. A cautious interpretation of the results really reveals nothing that was not already known, and the study did not set out to examine the relative merits of different models of supervision, failing to address the most important area of patient outcome. Because of the diverse nature of practice, the pooling of data may actually obfuscate specific findings. It is interesting to note that the application of clinical supervision in the various settings seems to have produced no detectable changes in measures of stress or job satisfaction in nurses.

Wolsey and Leach (1997) and Rogers (1998) have said that we have yet to show which models of clinical supervision are effective and, indeed, in which domains, for example patient outcome, nurse job satisfaction, etc., supervision makes a difference (Porter, 1988). One needs to bear in mind that, on the basis of the data we report in our study, 1 hour per month per nurse of one-to-one clinical supervision will mean the loss of one whole nurse for every 80 nurses employed. Over the country as a whole, this is a large commitment.

Like the motherhood and apple pie caricature, clinical supervision seems a good thing; however, the problem at the moment is that our knowledge of what works is to say the least sparse, and if we are to support such a massive investment in the future, some basic research questions need to be asked.

Background to clinical supervision in the Caswell Clinic

Clinical supervision for forensic mental health nurses is an under-reported and meagrely studied area despite writers having attempted to argue the need for clinical supervision when working with MDOs (Rogers and Topping-Morris, 1996). Our initial attempts at developing clinical supervision were focused on developing the right cultural base, by which clinical supervision was encouraged and fostered. It soon became apparent, however, that this alone was not sufficient to ensure that clinical supervision 'took hold'. Accordingly, a review of where we stood in terms of clinical supervision took place approximately 3 years ago. This review found that, whilst there was a positive attitude to the philosophy of clinical supervision, only a few were comfortable with knowing what, where and how they should go about this activity.

The principles of the nursing process underpin the activity of nursing within the Caswell Clinic, with a strong emphasis on collaboratively agreed care plans. The nursing process as a model is a problem-orientated approach to care. Nursing is often called upon to be problem orientated (Berger, 1984; Gournay, 1995; Hurst et al, 1991; McCarthy, 1981; Roberts et al, 1993; Rogers and Topping-Morris, 1997; Tanner et al, 1987; Taylor, 1997). Problem-orientated models of care and intervention have a sound basis for the activity of nursing. At present, the long postregistration ENB course (ENB 650) equips nurses to deliver problem-orientated behavioural psychotherapy (Marks, 1985). The 'Thorn' initiative (Gamble, 1995) – now more commonly referred to as psychosocial intervention training – focuses on problem-orientated care for families and sufferers of schizophrenia.

One of the writers had previously been seconded to the ENB 650 course (Adult Behavioural Psychotherapy) at the Institute of Psychiatry, London. A major theme running throughout this course is the process and skills involved in clinical supervision using a behavioural problem-focused approach. We therefore decided to develop a problem-orientated model of clinical supervision that, it was hoped, would ensure both a pragmatic and a flexible means of working.

Problem-orientated clinical supervision

Problem-orientated clinical supervision is a collaborative process wherein both supervisor and supervisee assess and identify clinical problems, and thereafter utilise the tenets of problem-solving strategies to ensure a structured, focused, logical and measurable means of finding solutions. It requires a collaborative process by which the supervisor encourages and facilitates self-actualisation of the supervisee in generating and resolving problems. This occurs on a graded basis until the supervisee becomes proficient in using the process with minimal assistance, thereby ensuring a generalisation of skills development and a decreasing reliance on the supervisor. Both parties actively seek to increase supervisee autonomy and utilise means of measuring change. The absolute principle guiding this is that evidence-based practices (as opposed to opinion or historically based practices) are the building blocks of effective clinical supervision.

Taylor (1997) provides an overview of problem-solving in clinical nursing practice and suggests that 'The art of caregiving requires knowledge, skills and expertise and central to effective practice is the ability to problem solve during implementation of care'. However, the ability to problem-solve is not an integral part of nurse training. This ability is a skill that, like other skills, will improve with practice and support.

Characteristics and principles of problem-orientated clinical supervision

Problem-orientated clinical supervision has its roots firmly in the pragmatic application of behaviourism. A major problem in adopting behavioural approaches within forensic mental health is the historically negative image that it evokes. However, Rogers (1997), in a description of the development of a nurse behavioural psychotherapy service in forensic mental health service, shows that behavioural approaches have significantly moved on from earlier applications and now have much to offer clients and services. The characteristics and principles of problem-orientated clinical supervision are:

- problem orientation, the supervisor and supervisee clearly identifying the problem clinical areas in terms of current, observed behaviour, thereafter developing systematic strategies to find solutions;

- structured short- and long-term goals for supervision and working towards these in a progressive manner;
- the supervisee being expected to be an active participant in clinical supervision (unlike in some other models). Furthermore, the main focus of supervision is to help the supervisee to set his or her own targets by identifying what needs to be done by when, by whom and in what manner, and how and when it will be evaluated;
- collaboration, there being no managerial mandate involved, as the supervisory process must be a two-way process, both parties assuming responsibility and accountability for agreed targets;
- development, the supervisee gradually developing skills in the problem-solving process within a framework of clinical effectiveness and being gradually expected to generalise these principles to his or her current practice. For example, the supervisory process may at first specifically focus on problem identification skills, then the accurate description of problems, then the principles of brainstorming, and then the process of generating solutions, with the identification of the benefits/disbenefits of each option. Nurses proficient in the above techniques will be able to critique literature and accurately review evidence for discussion at supervision prior to its integration into practice.

A case example of clinical supervision

This is an example of clinical supervision in the earlier stages that demonstrates the area of 'problem identification'.

A supervisee identifies a problem as 'refusing medication'; this relates to her work as the primary nurse for a recently admitted client who is refusing all oral medication. The client has told the nurse that he is tormented by command hallucinations and is unable to resist these, cutting himself, every day, in response. The client refuses all medication. The reasons behind his refusals have not been fully explored. Because of the client's disturbed mental state and self-injurious behaviour a decision is taken to medicate him with intramuscular injections. The supervisee has developed a comprehensive care plan that includes what should be done to maintain the client's dignity and the safety when injections are administered. The supervisee asks for assistance as she does not know how the team can further assist the client at this stage.

The focus of supervision in this situation is not to provide answers but to help the supervisee to identify other ways in which to formulate the problem. The supervisee and supervisor agree that further information is needed about why the client refuses medication, and the process of how the supervisee will approach the topic – based on what is known of the client – is agreed. The outcome of this is that, after three attempts by the nurse to gain more information, the client informs the nurse that he is 'not mentally ill or schizophrenic' as 'he is not mad'.

The focus of the next supervision session is to help the supervisee in reformulating the problem of refusing medication because the supervisee has realised that this is not the problem but is a manifestation of the real problem; refusing medication is a consequence of the client's not believing that he suffers from a mental illness. Furthermore, the supervisee then recognises that a previous attempt by the client to abscond may be related to this as the client has not identified with the psychiatric diagnosis or treatment. Thus, the problem is reformulated as 'the client and the clinical team are not working in collaboration due to a lack of agreement about diagnosis and treatment'. The supervisee begins to brainstorm several possible interventions for this problem, including a search of the literature in fields pertaining to the process of educating clients about diagnosis, and to command hallucinations. Having reviewed the literature available, and organised evidence for effective approaches, the nurse arranges a meeting with the client and the clinical team to propose and discuss a reformulation and to review the contemporary care plan.

This case example provides some insight into how the principles of problem-orientated clinical supervision are put into practice. Further examples of this process have been described by Sullivan and Rogers (1997), who described a primary nurse's successful use of cognitive behavioural therapy, with the assistance of clinical supervision, with a client who was paranoid. Rogers and Gronow (1997) described the application of cognitive behavioural interventions with clients with problems of anger.

Management and resource issues

It was agreed between nurse clinicians and managers that all charge nurses and above (nurses remunerated at F grade and above) should be trained to be clinical supervisors, which was achieved by the end of 1996. Members of staff attended an in-house, 2-day skills-based workshop. The clinic now has a complement of 18 clinical supervisors. The registered nursing workforce is 50, so each clinical supervisor is not expected to provide supervision to more than five nurses.

Nurses are enabled to choose their own clinical supervisors from this pool of 18. Access to other forms of clinical supervision is available and is utilised, and such specialised forms include cognitive behavioural therapy, forensic psychotherapy, psychology and medicine. However, these activities are viewed as adjuncts to, rather than replacements for, nursing clinical supervision.

Whilst the training was effective and served its purpose to 'prime' the workforce, it soon became apparent that the workforce is dynamic and that new starters, in small numbers, will require training. A 2-day workshop is uneconomic and an inefficient way to learn for such small numbers, so a process of training for new clinical supervisors had to be arranged to enable new members of staff to take supervisory roles. The underpinning tenet of the approach adopted was personal responsibility, new starters being accountable for the acquisition of skills that were identified with them for development. Skills acquisition is embedded in a set of targets for attainment. These include: having had a minimum of 1 year of experience at functioning in the current role; the role of clinical supervisor being linked to that person's individual performance review; having experienced six clinical supervision sessions as a supervisee in the past year; and being able to describe the rationale for recording a clinical supervision contract and discuss in detail how this would be done in a supervision session. Once an individual staff member has attained the targets, a screening interview takes place that ascertains levels of skill and knowledge. Before the individual can begin supervising others, these steps must be successfully completed.

The cost of setting up a clinical supervision infrastructure is financially heavy. Our experience of providing clinical supervision for 43 identified nurses for 1 hour per month requires a total of 1032 hours of qualified nursing time. This is the equivalent of 20 hours of qualified nurse time per week. Owing to the large demand on the nursing resource (and the lack of persuasive evidence to date on the financial effectiveness of clinical supervision), we decided to evaluate the impact of clinical supervision through an audit of standards and a client satisfaction survey. Furthermore, we wanted to measure if our particular model of clinical supervision was being effective.

Evaluation through an audit of standards

The clinic has developed a local policy on the provision of clinical supervision. This policy identifies that an audit of clinical supervision will take place on a yearly basis. As reported elsewhere (Rogers and Topping-Morris, 1997), all nursing staff have been provided with an individual clinical supervision portfolio that contains the policy, the standards and audit protocol, the contract and session records. The audit method is by a review of these records. The sample for audit was selected at random, comprising 31% of the nursing staff. During the audit process, nurses were at liberty to indicate that their individual profiles were not used; no member of staff chose to do this.

The standards and outcomes

Measures were taken against the following standards:

1. All nurses engaged in clinical supervision will receive clinical supervision from an appropriately trained supervisor (Table 15.1).
2. All supervisors will negotiate a written contract with their supervisees (Table 15.2).
3. Clinical supervisor and supervisee will keep records of issues discussed in every supervision session using the agreed format for sessional record-keeping (Table 15.3).
4. Supervisor and supervisee will follow policy guidelines regarding the storage of supervision records (Table 15.4).
5. Clinical supervisors, using a problem-orientated approach, will assist the supervisee to devise action plans to meet the supervisee's requirements (Table 15.5).

Discussion

As the results of the audit demonstrate, the systems that are in place are ensuring that the majority of the supervisee's needs are being met. The most significant finding is that not all nurses are as yet engaging in monthly clinical supervision, one of the reasons for this being the employment of new staff. However, further analysis of the current staffing systems demonstrated that supervisees and supervisors were having to cancel sessions at short notice because of the immediate needs of the clients (for example, escorting patients on walks, the changing needs of clients' observation levels, rehabilitation activities, etc). We are therefore currently piloting a system of having a dedicated day each month when nursing clinical supervision is prioritorised and when nursing resources and the demands on such resources are carefully managed. This has involved enlisting the assistance of all clinical teams in preplanning the demands in terms of nurse escorting and clinical meetings for this day.

Table 15.1. Breakdown of nurses who have or have not registered with a clinical supervisor ($n = 45$)

	Total who have a clinical supervisor	% of sample	Total who do not have a clinical supervisor	% of sample
ALL AREAS	35	78	10	22

Table 15.2. 'All supervisors will negotiate a written contract with their supervisees' ($n = 13$)

	Number achieved	% Achieved
1. A written contract has been made of the content for clinical supervision	12	92
2. Both parties have signed the contract	11	77
3. Both parties maintain copies of the contract and bring them to each session	12	92
4. All aspects of supervision have been negotiated into the contract and recorded	12	92

Table 15.3. 'Clinical supervisor and supervisee will keep records of issues discussed in every supervision session using the agreed format for sessional record-keeping' ($n = 13$)

	Number achieved	% Achieved
1. A signed record of each session is maintained by both supervisor and supervisee	12	92
2. Supervisor and supervisee bring records to each session	12	92
3. Terms of contract for keeping records have been followed	12	92
4. Supervisee and supervisor have agreed on content of records	12	92

Table 15.4. 'Supervisor and supervisee will follow policy guidelines regarding the storage of supervision records' ($n = 13$)

	Number achieved	% Achieved
1. Both parties have discussed issues of confidentiality and breaches of confidentiality	13	100
2. Written contract has included issues of confidentiality and the breaching of confidentiality	13	100
3. Both parties have agreed on when confidentiality is to be breached	13	100
4. Both parties follow the policy on confidentiality of records	13	100

Table 15.5. 'Clinical supervisors, using a problem-orientated approach, will assist the supervisee in devising action plans to meet the supervisee's requirements' ($n = 13$)

	Number achieved	% Achieved
1. Clinical supervisor uses a problem-solving approach to facilitate the devising of action plans to meet the supervisee's clinical need	13	100
2. Action plans are in evidence in supervision records	12	92

Our experiences to date have challenged our original views that clinical supervision will occur simply through increased awareness and organisational agreement alone. So far, the systems we have had to develop include:

• providing staff training;
• developing the necessary documentation records;
• developing a policy;
• setting and auditing standards;
• managing our available resources.

It is not known whether these systems will be specifically needed in developing clinical supervision for all nurses, whether our experience is unique in so far as forensic mental health nurses are usually working in inpatient environments, and/or whether it is affected by the population served and the need for a flexible nursing workforce.

Finally, whilst it appears that clinical supervision is now occurring within a framework of systems that allow us to collect evaluative data and develop new ideas about this complex process, we were also concerned that our adopted model of problem-orientated clinical supervision was satisfying our staff. One of our major goals in developing this model of clinical supervision was not to ensure that it happens because a number of reports state that it should, but to meet effectively the needs of the nursing staff, who in this circumstance are our customers. To this effect, we have also conducted a review of the model through the use of a supervision satisfaction survey.

Evaluation of clinical supervisee satisfaction

Our second goal was to evaluate how useful our model of clinical supervision was to supervisees. The sample used to measure the satisfaction with clinical supervision was all the qualified nurses on permanent contracts of employment whose nursing role was predominantly focused on direct clinical intervention and care. The sample did not include those nurses who were on temporary contracts or those whose role was predominantly managerial or educational in focus.

At the time of the survey, the Caswell Clinic employed 50 registered nurses. Of these, 43 were employed in permanent clinical positions, in which clinical supervision was identified as an essential aspect of clinical nursing practice. All of these nurses had the option of not engaging in clinical supervision, but none took this up.

Of the remaining 7 staff who were not sent questionnaires, 2 were employed on a temporary basis. The remaining 5 were employed in managerial or educational posts and did not need clinical supervision; they did, however, receive managerial supervision. The satisfaction levels of these staff is not included in this report.

Method

There are many problems in choosing an instrument for measuring satisfaction. Ricketts (1996) provides an excellent summary of these issues as identified by other writers. Problems with reported studies (into client satisfaction) were identified by Lebow (1982) to be in three main areas. First, many studies developed their own instruments, often without any report on validation, rendering a comparison of satisfaction rates across different studies impossible. Second, client sampling is open to possible bias from two sources: client selection and response rates. Third, the high degree of satisfaction reported in many studies where a single measure was taken is meaningless in the absence of either comparison between centres or repeated measurement over time. Parloff (1983) argues that many satisfaction surveys, in the absence of comparative data, were simply performing a public relations function.

A review of the literature demonstrated that the majority of evaluative studies on clinical supervision have used different measures (for example, the General Health Questionnaire or job satisfaction questionnaires) to assess outcomes. However, many have focused on concepts such as the mental health, stress, burn-out, coping skills and job satisfaction of responders. These measures are significantly flawed as they do not control for extraneous variables outside clinical supervision, which can affect the items being measured. For example, Butterworth et al (1997) used the General Health Questionnaire and the Harris Nurse Stress Index in an evaluative study of clinical supervision and mentorship commissioned by both the Department of Health and the Scottish Home and Health Department. Both of these measures are designed to identify stress symptoms in the respondent. This method of evaluating clinical supervision (through the psychological state of the respondent) does not necessarily consider that work is but one area contributing to a person's stress. Consequently, the conclusions that can be drawn from such data lack generalisability and cannot be attributed solely to one variable (clinical supervision).

For this reason, the instrument used to evaluate the effect of clinical supervision was a slightly modified version of the Client Satisfaction Questionnaire (CSQ) as devised by Larsen et al (1979). Written permission was given for some slight modification of the wording of this instrument in order to relate it to clinical supervision. Ricketts (1996) provides a summary of the CSQ:

> The CSQ was developed by Larsen and colleagues and relates to the construct of general satisfaction as the 'undifferentiated positive regard for outcome. The CSQ consists of eight items scored on a 1-4 scale, with 4 indicating maximum

satisfaction. Since development, the CSQ has been utilized extensively in the USA as a reliable means of measuring a consumer's satisfaction with the service that they have received.

Whilst there are a number of problems in our use of this measurement, namely those identified by Lebow (1982), we decided to use this measure as it is an established method of measuring satisfaction and because we wanted to pilot its usefulness as a measure of satisfaction with clinical supervision.

The identified sample group were all sent questionnaires and asked to complete them within 3 weeks. A reminder was sent to all staff who had not returned their questionnaires, asking them to complete them within a further 3 weeks. The questionnaire asked respondents basic demographic questions: name, grade and work area. They were then asked to answer eight 'set' questions and indicate their answer on a 4-point scale. Confidentiality was emphasised in order to maximise compliance with the study and the truthfulness of the respondents.

Results

Forty-three questionnaires were distributed, 25 of which were returned, representing a response rate of 58%. Of the 25 respondents, 4 were not receiving clinical supervision, which means that the data from 21 respondents were used in the analysis. Data from the tables below show the following:

- Table 15.6, the respondents' gender;
- Table 15.7, their grades;
- Table 15.8, the respondents' rating of the quality of the clinical supervision received;
- Table 15.9, the level of supervision wanted;
- Table 15.10, whether the clinical supervision mode or model met their needs;
- Table 15.11, whether the model would be recommended to others;
- Table 15.12, the respondents' satisfaction rating;
- Table 15.13, their rating regarding clinical supervision enhancing clinical effectiveness;
- Table 15.14, their overall satisfaction rating;
- Table 15.15, the likelihood of the model being used again by the supervisees.

Table 15.6. Gender of respondents $(n = 25)$

	Number of respondents	% Of sample
Male	12	48
Female	13	52

Table 15.7. Grade of respondents

	Number of respondents	% Of sample
Grade D	1	4
Grade E	15	60
Grade F	6	24
Grade G	3	12

Table 15.8. Respondents' rating of the quality of the clinical supervision $(n = 21)$

	Total	Percentage
Excellent	8	38
Good	10	48
Fair	3	14
Poor	0	0

Table 15.9. Respondents' ratings of whether they received the clinical supervision they wanted $(n = 21)$

	Total	Percentage
Definitely not	0	0
Not really	0	0
Generally yes	15	71
Definitely yes	6	29

Table 15.10. Respondents' ratings of whether the model met their needs $(n = 21)$

	Total	Percentage
Almost all of my needs are met	4	19
Most of my needs are met	16	76
Only a few of my needs are met	1	5
None of my needs is met	0	0

Table 15.11. Respondents' ratings of whether they recommend the model to others ($n = 21$)

	Total	Percentage
Definitely not	0	0
Not really	0	0
Generally yes	15	71
Definitely yes	6	29

Table 15.12. Respondents' ratings of satisfaction ($n = 21$)

	Total	Percentage
Quite dissatisfied	1	5
Indifferent or mildly dissatisfied	0	0
Mostly satisfied	16	76
Very satisfied	4	19

Table 15.13. Respondents' ratings of clinical effectiveness ($n = 21$)

	Total	Percentage
Yes, it's helped a great deal	4	19
Yes, it's helped somewhat	17	81
No, it didn't help	0	0
No, it made things worse	0	0

Table 15.14. Respondents' ratings of overall satisfaction ($n = 21$)

	Total	Percentage
Quite dissatisfied	0	0
Indifferent or mildly dissatisfied	4	19
Mostly satisfied	12	57
Very satisfied	5	24

Table 15.15. Respondents' ratings of whether they would use this model in the future ($n = 21$)

	Total	Percentage
No, Definitely not	0	0
No, I don't think so	2	9
Yes, I think so	14	67
Yes, definitely	5	24

Discussion

The instrument used allows for a comparison between general satisfaction and general dissatisfaction through a comparison of positive
or negative responses for all questions (Table 15.16). Larsen et al
(1979) suggest that focusing on dissatisfaction data may be one way
to make satisfaction surveys more useful to providers who are trying
to improve their services. All respondents had the opportunity to
provide positive or negative comments at the end of the questionnaire. The negative responses are drawn up in Figure 15.1.

This study into audit and satisfaction has highlighted a number of
issues related to clinical supervision at the Caswell Clinic. There is
one major limitation of this study, which must be considered in so far
as the instruments chosen do not allow for a comparison across time
or across different sites at this stage. However, as this is our first
comprehensive review, this will change with time, and we will be able
to examine trends across time. On a positive note, the instruments
we used have managed to measure exactly what they were intended
to: whether our standards are being met and whether supervisees are
satisfied with the model adopted.

Overall, the evaluative study achieved its aims, which were to
evaluate clinical supervision as it stands at present and to evaluate
whether our model is acceptable to supervisees. Clinical supervision
is a very difficult process to audit and measure; there is little evidence
available in the literature that allows for comparisons across different
sites. The problem-orientated model that we have adopted appears
to have been widely accepted by the majority of staff. The original
aim was to develop a model that would meet the needs of most of the
people most of the time, as it was felt that no one universal model
currently existed. When clinical supervision happens, it is focused
and problem orientated, develops clear actions for supervisees to
achieve and focuses on clinical care, treatment and management.

It is also intended to introduce more rigorous means of rating
both the problems and targets identified, and an evaluation of clinical supervision between supervisee and supervisor. It is feasible that

Table 15.16. Satisfied or dissatisfied? ($n = 168$)

	Total	Percentage
Positive responses	157	93
Negative responses	11	7

Resources

- There are often difficulties ensuring appointments are met due to unexpected difficulties in resource needs
- It continues to be difficult to arrange times and dates for supervision, particularly if one has been arranged, and for example, I am the only qualified nurse on duty
- I feel that not all people are utilising clinical supervision, although this is not a reflection on the supervision model
- My first supervisor and I would plan a date and time; however clinical needs would step in and replace it. My supervisor then transferred to another ward. My second supervisor is part time and co-ordinating dates and times has proved difficult
- On a personal level, my current supervisor has moved wards and I haven't had a supervision session recently. However, they are to resume shortly. I feel that clinical supervision has been beneficial to my practice and for my confidence when dealing with difficult problems
- To elaborate on my mildly dissatisfied answer, which I am sure is a 'bug bear' for many people, is arranging the date and then finding out that due to resources throughout the unit the session needs to be cancelled
- Due to staffing levels, I find that planned supervision sessions have to be cancelled on occasions. I would like a system where time is allocated for such sessions and fitted in where possible

The model

- I have found that there is definitely an emphasis on supervision [at Caswell] that I have not seen before in generic mental health practice. The problem-orientated approach provides a clear distinction between interpreting behaviours and implementing care. I personally require two systems where I am able to gain insight into how my behaviour affects care as well as problem solving. I would welcome being taught how to supervise others using the problem-orientated approach
- Once you've mastered the problem-solving approach, most can do it independently of the supervisor. What is important is the supervisor's skill in helping the supervisee to explore and examine different solutions which they may not have thought of
- I feel that different approaches help me to develop my clinical skills and ways of thinking. I feel reasonably confident in the problem-solving process, and I am able to work through this process independently

Figure 15.1. Comments relating to resources and models.

this could be done using the problems and target measurements (Marks et al, 1986) used by behaviour nurse therapists in everyday clinical practice. This would allow further evaluation of the effectiveness in problem reduction through our model.

Conclusions

This chapter has provided an overview of the development and evaluation of clinical supervision for forensic mental health nurses in one

MSU. When we began this venture, we did not expect the difficulties we would encounter with regard to the amount of time, resources, structure and problems that we encountered. Nevertheless, our experience is that this development is providing our staff and clients with many clinical benefits, which we are unable clearly to evidence at this time. We intend to conduct a further study on whether agreed action plans developed in clinical supervision are put into clinical practice. Then we will be better able to evaluate whether the process of clinical supervision is making a real difference to clinical care and to our clients.

Acknowledgements

The Client Satisfaction Questionnaire © (CSQ) modified for Clinical Supervision was developed at the University of California San Francisco by Drs Clifford Attkisson and Daniel Larsen in collaboration with Drs William A. Hargreaves, Maurice LeVois, Tuan Nguyen, Robert E. Roberts and Bruce Stegner. Copyright © 1979, 1989, 1990. Used with the written permission of Clifford Attkisson, PhD.

References

Berger MC (1984) Clinical thinking ability and nursing students. Journal of Nursing Education 23(7): 306–8.

Butterworth T, Carson J, White E, Jeacock J, Clements A, Bishop V (1997) It is good to talk: an evaluation of clinical supervision and mentorship in England and Scotland. Manchester: University of Manchester.

Department of Health (1994) Working in Partnership: Report of the Review of Mental Health Nursing. London: Department of Health.

Gamble C (1995) The Thorn nurse training initiative. Nursing Standard 9(15): 31–4.

Gournay K (1995) Mental health nurses working purposefully with people with serious and enduring mental illness – an international perspective. International Journal of Nursing Studies 4: 341–52.

Hurst K, Sean A, Trickey S (1991) The recognition and non-recognition of problem-solving strategies in nursing practice. Journal of Advanced Nursing 16: 1444–55.

Larsen DL, Attkisson CC, Hargreaves WA, Nguyen TD (1979) Assessment of client/patient satisfaction: development of a general scale. Evaluation and Program Planning 2: 197–207.

Lebow J (1982) Consumer satisfaction with mental health treatment. Psychological Bulletin 91: 244–59.

McCarthy MM (1981) The nursing process: application of current thinking in clinical problem solving. Journal of Advanced Nursing 6: 173–7.

Marks IM (1985) Psychiatric Nurse Therapists in Primary Care. London: Royal College of Nursing.

Marks IM, Bird J, Brown M, Ghost A (1986) Behavioural Psychotherapy: Maudsley

Pocket Book of Clinical Management. Bristol: John Wright.

NHS Management Executive (1993) A Vision for the Future: The Nursing, Midwifery and Health Visiting Contribution to Health Care. London: Department of Health.

Parloff MB (1983) Who will be satisfied by consumer satisfaction evidence? Behaviour Therapy 14: 242–6.

Porter N (1998) Providing effective clinical supervision. Nursing Management 5(2): 22–3.

Ricketts T (1996) General satisfaction and satisfaction with nursing communication on an adult psychiatric ward. Journal of Advanced Nursing 24: 479–84.

Roberts JD, While AE, Fitzpatrick JM (1993) Problem solving in nursing practice: application, process, skill acquisition and measurement. Journal of Advanced Nursing 18: 886–91.

Rogers P (1997) Behaviour nurse therapy in forensic mental health. Mental Health Practice 1(4): 22–6.

Rogers P (1998) Hype that is hard to swallow. Mental Health Practice 1(10): 18.

Rogers P, Gronow T (1997) Turning down the heat. Nursing Times 93(43): 26–9.

Rogers P, Topping-Morris B (1996) Prison and the role of the forensic mental health nurse. Nursing Times 92(31): 32–4.

Rogers P, Topping-Morris B (1997) Clinical supervision for forensic mental health nurses. Nursing Management 4(5): 13–15.

Royal College of Psychiatrists (1996) The Report of the Confidential Inquiry into Homicides and Suicides by Mentally Ill People. London: Royal College of Psychiatrists.

Sullivan J, Rogers P (1997) Cognitive behavioural nursing therapy in paranoid psychosis. Nursing Times 93(2): 28–30.

Tanner CA, Padrick K, Westfall U, Putzier D (1987) Diagnostic reasoning strategies of nurses and nursing students. Nursing Research 36(6): 358–63.

Taylor C (1997) Problem solving in clinical nursing practice. Journal of Advanced Nursing 26: 329–36.

UKCC (United Kingdom Central Council for Nursing, Midwifery and Health Visiting) (1994) The Future of Professional Practice – the UKCC's Standards for Education and Practice Following Registration. London: UKCC.

Welsh Office (1996) Caring for the Future: The Nursing Agenda for Mental Health Nursing Action Plan. Cardiff: Welsh Office.

Wolsey P, Leach L (1997) Clinical supervision: a hornet's nest? Nursing Times 93(44): 24–7.

Chapter 16
Developing the contribution of research in nursing: accessing the state-of-the-art in technology and information

DAVID ROBINSON

There is an abundance of research texts that more than adequately describe the elements of the research process, citing many examples. It is the intention of this author not to repeat what has been published but to offer something new. Forensic psychiatric care offers its own discrete challenges, and the process of carrying out research is just the same. This chapter offers a more informative approach; it identifies that adopting a research method does not necessarily mean that rigorous scientific experimental designs need be used. Research is about using information to influence one's ideas and is not just about finding answers to hypotheses.

This chapter, therefore, discusses some of the challenges facing nurses and identifies some of the current nursing-led innovations that can be used to establish and disseminate new knowledge. Furthermore, it will open up new horizons, offering the reader new avenues and resources to explore and gain new skills and knowledge.

Implementing practitioner research

The benefits of research within forensic services have been well documented (Taylor, 1991); also, research programmes may provide a unique opportunity to bring caring disciplines together through collaborative programmes that ultimately lead to new knowledge – and improved patient care. Smith (1986) addressed nurses in terms relevant to many practitioner groups when he urged the profession to implement research findings and stated that most research reports contain at least one finding that could be implemented on the wards. If we are to contribute to the improvement of practice through research and the application of its findings, the prime objective is to ensure that research and development (R&D) becomes an integral part of health care (Department of Health, 1991a, 1992a, 1993a, 1993b).

Sheehan (1986) noted that applying research findings in clinical practice is the biggest challenge facing nurses wishing to undertake research. Implementing research in practice is a demanding task requiring rigour and discipline as well as creativity, clinical judgement and skill (Webb and Mackenzie, 1993). It is important to dispel the myth that every practitioner should carry out research – although all should use elements of the research process in developing a questioning and evaluative approach to care.

Professional practice as research based

A major function of practitioner research is to strengthen the knowledge bases of the health professions and thus enhance clinical performance (Marsland, 1993). Darling and Rodgers (1986) have discussed the health professions' need to confirm their role as research based and have concluded that this is being attempted. Systematic enquiry into all aspects of care is necessary to defend decisions on a scientific basis, rather than simply on an intuitive or conventional one (Clark and Hockey, 1979). This must be the case if nurses are to satisfy the legal requirement related to their professional practice that their actions are based upon the most recently available factual knowledge (UKCC, 1993).

One criterion put forward as essential to a profession is the possession of a specific body of knowledge, and a major route to acquiring this is through research. The past decade has seen a considerable increase in the number of research-based health care publications, yet little as yet has been published within the field of forensic mental health nursing research. Similarly, until recently, there have been few attempts to bring research and good practice together in a concentrated way that allows people to access the latest information on a given subject.

Although organisational change has been rapid, related changes in clinical practice have been ponderously slow. Taking steps to ensure that care practice is based upon theories that are formulated and verified scientifically will ultimately increase the body of knowledge, improve caring skills and promote the quality of health care. In a climate of quality and cost-effectiveness, health care research is essential if standards are to be verified and if care offered to patients is to be based upon the best available information and resources. Nurses need to obtain verifiable data that will influence decision-making and policies in a cost-effective manner. If they do not grasp the importance of research in this respect, it is certain that other professionals will seek to do it for them.

It appears, on the face of it, that, apart from a few prolific writers, research and related developmental programmes rarely get into print, which would indicate that there is little development at ward level. This is clearly not the case as, within my own visits to units and wards, I have seen many dynamic staff working within innovative programmes. These programmes are frequently reported via news releases or in-house communications. For example in 1995, the Special Hospitals Service Authority, in collaboration with the Department of Health, published a book of abstracts relating to achievements against the Vision for the Future targets (Department of Health and Special Hospitals Service Authority, 1995). Whilst this represented effective dissemination, few of these programmes were subsequently published in full. There are training and development (and more often than not time) issues in writing for publication, but practitioners have to get to grips with publishing and disseminating more widely if we are to develop the profession and our body of knowledge.

Nurses have a unique opportunity to develop care practices and influence the future development of health care (Department of Health, 1993a). The collection and use of scientific data enables them to define the parameters of their profession and describe its unique contribution to health care. It can also determine the effectiveness of professional actions, help to develop theoretical frameworks and ensure more informed decision-making in daily practice. Without thinking about it, the nurse is inevitably involved in at least some stage of the research process within his or her daily activities and is ideally placed to carry out research (Brooks, 1988; Reed and Dean, 1986). In support of other professionals, nurses may play a vital role in bringing nursing's perspective to the enrichment of collaborative research programmes. By virtue of the long periods that nurses spend in attending to patients' needs, they are uniquely placed to offer valuable insights into problems of patient care and to influence treatment.

Encouraging developmental change

There is a need to encourage developmental changes within practitioner research in forensic care so that it is no longer principally reliant on individuals offering well-developed programmes, usually expressed through enrolments on research courses (although these will continue to play an important part). There are still few posts dedicated to full-time research that both have academic validity and possess adequate resources. Subjectively, nurses have been criticised for their supposed obsession with research into nursing practice to the exclusion of more consumer-orientated programmes. The R&D strategy (Department of Health, 1993b) clearly identifies such research as a valid part of nursing evaluation, although there is, perhaps, a need to redress the balance by involving nurses and other health care professionals in ensuring that research activity is geared to patient need, to demonstrating cost-effectiveness and to attaining organisational objectives.

The past 5 years have seen a growth in nursing research programmes within the forensic psychiatric hospitals. Within high secure services, there have been over 70 studies carried out at various levels – those of the diploma, first degree, Master's and PhD. In addition, there are many examples of good practice and innovation occurring that could be the seeds of R&D programmes. Clinical nurse specialists and nurses who have completed related research courses should be centrally involved in developing appropriate research programmes, especially within their own work areas. Similarly, these 'resource' persons should be key people in developing a climate supportive to enquiry and evaluation. Obviously, if R&D is to be credible, appropriate academic support and supervision must be maintained. Research cannot afford to continue unco-ordinated; it requires to be managed in a supportive environment.

Action research programmes can involve individual nurses in systematic enquiry with members of other disciplines, without distancing them from clinical practice. Experienced researchers can foster and develop these programmes, provide supervisory support, ensure credibility and help to disseminate results to bridge the theory–practice gap. Furthermore, nurses can help to supply the frequently missing link by testing out and validating already existing research findings in practice. These issues were illustrated in a discussion with research students who were divided in their views. Half of the group clearly felt that educational courses helped them to understand the research process and enabled them to spread the gospel of research to colleagues. The other half felt that 'research jargon' distanced them from colleagues and resulted in support for the élitist impression of research.

Demystification of research as an élitist activity

A demystification of research at clinical level is essential, and a practical demonstration and growth of research activity needs to be fostered in close relationship to the living contexts of everyday care. Although there are numerous publications and locally produced handouts that set out to introduce health practitioners to research, these frequently assume a working knowledge of the 'research vocabulary' and often introduce more terminology without clarifying any of it. Meanwhile, the growing number of research reports, theses and journal articles themselves introduce more and more terms, which adds to the feeling of being perplexed. Research reports, especially those originating from unfamiliar disciplines, can alienate health carers because of their specialised presentation. Generally speaking, writers on research have only recently begun to 'translate' research terms and findings meaningfully and understandably for the practitioner. Clarity is required if we are to move towards a research-based profession and adopt evidence-based care and clinical effectiveness.

De-jargonising jargon

Research textbooks frequently offer glossaries explaining specific research terms. However, these are rarely exhaustive and tend to be written for the initiated rather than the novice. Research terms require careful presentation in order to overcome unnecessary semantic barriers. *The A to Z of Social Research Jargon* (Robinson and Reed, 1998) addresses these issues. The main aim of this text is to help break down the barriers (unintentionally) erected by academic writers and thus explain key issues in accessible language. It contains almost 300 terms and is written to provide insight into research vocabulary. It will allow those already familiar with basic terms further to explore some related concepts, and it will foster creative curiosity and the desire to read further. The editors have taken into account issues stressed by many health practitioners, and the resultant text has been carefully structured to offer the reader at all levels examples of terms and definitions in a handy format. A typical entry will include the following:

- *Term.* Many of these are terms used in everyday research. There are also some terms that, whilst not exclusive to research, are certainly relevant since they deal with related subjects such as ethics, philosophy and informatics.
- *Everyday use.* The colloquial or 'ordinary language' origin of a research term is given to provide the background from which it has acquired its special use. This is a short lay explanation with meaningfulness as its first aim.
- *Research use.* Here, the stipulative definition used by researchers is given. This enables the reader to compare 'ordinary language' with research versions. Equating everyday with research usage is an important step in learning research terms.
- *Example.* Here, practical research example(s) are offered to help the reader to establish how technology is used. Descriptions of practical research in action have been chosen to reflect frequently occurring situations often encountered by health carers in the contexts of their daily work.
- *Related terms.* These are listed to highlight terms usually associated with the key term. Detailed definitions of these can be found elsewhere in the text.

Developing managerial and organisational commitment

Nurse managers play an important role in the research process as they promote cost-effectiveness in health care delivery. One way to justify this is through research. Unless managers understand the contribution that research can make to the organisation and clinical practice, naiveté will dominate. The major changes promulgated for the service for MDOs will need to draw on systematic evaluation if managers are to provide evidence of enhanced quality and value for money.

Ward managers especially may exert influence in developing care skills and are well placed to develop research-based care. They could, for example, facilitate the emergence of the 'nurse scientist'. For example, nurses' time may be allocated to review the literature, to look at other examples of good practice related to patient need and to evaluate how practice may be changed and improved. Individualised care programming based upon the latter process should result in improved outcomes for patients.

All managers within the organisation should have research objectives as integral parts of their roles; these may include dissemination through conferences and journal publications. Organisational commitment must be developed if a research-based culture in nursing and other disciplines is to germinate. Research must be firmly placed upon the agenda of all managers as they are required to seek solutions to problems. Decision-makers within the organisation need to identity areas where R&D is most likely to benefit patients, staff and the organisation. Similarly, managers and nurses need to identify and use the results of research to ensure that practice is dynamic. Ward and other managers are key persons in targeting appropriate education and training, enabling them to foster and develop research programmes and create a climate supportive to the questioning and evaluation of practice, Also, they are uniquely placed to identify priority issues for further R&D activity.

Research priorities

Local and national research priorities have been well documented (see, for example, Department of Health, 1992a, 1993a, 1993b; Grubin and Gunn, 1991; Rae, 1994; Reed, 1992; Reed and Robinson, 1992; Taylor, 1991). A review by the Special Hospitals Service Authority (1993a) revealed that approximately 35% of ward managers felt that little of their current ward-based practice was based upon contemporary research findings. However, they identified numerous research projects (some of which were in hand), although no details were provided regarding the level of such investigations. Projects thought necessary included the assessment of dangerousness, alternatives to seclusion, control and restraint, deliberate self-harm, the treatment of sex offenders, primary nursing and various topics relating to the patient as a consumer of care; some of these were recommended by the Blackwood Report (Special Hospitals Service Authority, 1993b).

Whilst projects were identified, little evidence could be found of the dissemination of known knowledge, which illustrates the requirement to circulate details of recently completed (and ongoing) R&D. Research and good practice must be disseminated if practice is to develop.

Informing practice

One of the core issues in facilitating research is how best to promote the ability to 'find out how to find out'; here information sources are invaluable. This brings into the debate the importance of networking locally and throughout the NHS and knowing where to find information. Whilst some information sources have been well developed over the years, they have been limited to traditional research centres and are often in inaccessible places. Substantial effort is needed to develop NHS networking if R&D is to be integrated. More emphasis on communication and the dissemination of good practice is required throughout hospitals and the NHS, as well as within hospitals. Sharing good practice through R&D forums is of the essence in promoting quality health care. Specialty forums on clinically important topics (for example, issues relating to self-harm) are needed to make research-based findings accessible to clinically based staff.

The Institute of Psychiatry has created an International Register of forensic research (Grubin and Gunn, 1991), with a view to publishing a yearly update. This is a useful way in which to identify what is available, although it falls short of identifying research in nursing (few nurse researchers being identified). This may be because the author exclusively identifies studies that are directly related to the care of the MDO. Studies that are indirectly related (for example, Heber, 1987; Mogg et al, 1987; Roberson, 1992) could also be useful. The International Register is an important resource that could provide nurses with extremely useful information on many aspects of MDO research. Indeed, the Register provides a directory of specialised expertise that may be utilised by all disciplines. There are other resources – well established and valuable (although underused) – that indicate research-based activity and information: the Cochrane database, Psyclit, Cenal, the Steinberg collection of research at the Royal College of Nursing, and the Network for Psychiatric Nursing Research database at Oxford. All require more development in relation to forensic care.

The International Forensic Psychiatric Database

The dissemination of R&D knowledge has been confined to publications and conference participation, and many programmes are unknown because developments are rarely brought together. Butterworth (1994) suggested the development of information sources that are accessible by nurses within their workplace. The International Forensic Psychiatric Database has been created to promote the dissemination of research findings and enhance practice. The recent development of this database to identify programmes for dissemination has resulted in an international initiative allowing more sharing and access of knowledge.

National Forensic Nurses' Research and Development Group

In 1991, a national R&D forum was developed by nurses engaged in research in the three English Special Hospitals (Ashworth, Broadmoor and Rampton) and the State Hospital, Carstairs, Scotland. Supported by the Special Hospitals Service Authority, the forum was a subgroup of its Nursing Development Group. The intention was to inform the leaders of nursing about key research issues. The forum's aims included support for nurses undertaking research within these hospitals, the dissemination of research findings, establishing a research network and identifying key areas for future research programmes. The forum was successful in organising a regular Networking Newsletter to communicate good practice and R&D. In addition, the forum was instrumental in facilitating two conferences on innovations in forensic services, which celebrated good practice.

Whilst the nursing R&D forum networked within the wider NHS, the group's activities were mainly directed towards promoting R&D within the Special Hospitals. The forum's final aim within the auspices of the Special Hospitals Service Authority was to integrate its activities within the wider NHS. This wider, NHS-integrated group was to be a new venture in R&D networking, representing all branches of forensic nursing on a UK basis.

Following the successful identification to and confirmation of members in the new group, a series of meetings was held prior to its official launch on 24 October 1996 at a multiprofessional forensic conference in Nottingham. The new National Forensic Nurses' Research and Development Group included people involved in research and related research activities. Members of the group offer a wide range of experiences from prisons, high-security services, medium and low secure provision, psychiatric intensive care units and community and university settings. The group was careful to foster strong links with universities and academic programmes, and included three PhD holders within the inaugural group's membership. The aims and objectives of the group are of particular relevance to nurses and other staff in generic and specialist settings who work with MDOs. Aims include:

- to promote the contribution of nursing in the R&D of forensic mental health care in a wider multidisciplinary context;
- to establish and contribute to a body of knowledge to inform practice.

The objectives include:

- identifying contacts in all forensic and related services for the purposes of two-way communication, both nationally and internationally;
- identifying and promoting current research and good practice;
- establishing channels of dissemination/communication through the Internet and the NHS Centre for Reviews and Dissemination at the University of York (CRD).

How would the National Forensic Nurses' Group link with others?

Collecting information about R&D is of little use if there is no recognised mechanism for its dissemination. A number of initiatives were explored, including forensic newsletters, supplements and conferences/seminars. During this exploration, the CRD was identified as a potential collaborator. The CRD is a national centre for reviews and dissemination, its role being to promote the use of research-based knowledge in health care. Subsequently, the International Forensic Psychiatric Database was linked by the National Forensic Nurses' Research and Development Group to the CRD initiative. There have been three key players in the development of this database:

- Rampton Hospital Authority have committed resources through the involvement of R&D staff who provide central data collection and input to the master database.
- The National Forensic Nurses' Research and Development Group provides local resources to promote the database and to encourage participants to register their initiatives. The group also provides national networking through regular meetings and newsletters to monitor progress. Conferences throughout the country also contribute to major networking.
- The Practice and Service Development Initiative (PSDI) at the University of York – a project based at the CRD – is focused upon the research needs of the nursing and therapy professions. They provide the resources for support to copy and disseminate the database nationally.

The CRD had for some time been profiling R&D activities across the regions, five of which had been profiled. Although hundreds of R&D initiatives were identified, only 17 were from the forensic mental health care sector; it was clear that there was a huge gap. CRD profiling has always been multiprofessional, and the National Forensic Nurses' Research and Development Group were committed to supporting this: thus, the word 'nurses' was deleted from explanatory letters and data collection schedules.

Data collection

Since detailed data collection had been successful within the CRD regional profiles, it was important to utilise the instrument in its current format with only minor modifications to accommodate forensic aspects. This was done, through piloting, using a multiprofessional sample. Key questions from the questionnaire are outlined in Figure 16.1. Covering letters explaining the initiative, along with the questionnaires, were distributed to forensic units across the UK, as well as to community and university areas. In addition, international mailings were targeted, being identified through various registers and publications. A total of 350 questionnaires were distributed. Data collection and input at Rampton Hospital covered the period July to November 1997.

Name:
Contact Address:
Telephone: **Fax:**
E-Mail:

In which area of health care is your place of work?:
What is your profession?:
What are your roles within that profession?:
Is this practice development/clinical effectiveness:
- Funded
- Research based
- Multidisciplinary
- Directly affecting patients
- A development in the delivery of services?
- Are outcome measures being used in this practice/service development?

Topic area of work:
Patient group:
Areas in which this work is being undertaken:
Are you undertaking this piece of work in collaboration with others?:
Please describe your work in as much detail as you can:
Would you find it useful to receive research-based information regarding your topic area of work?:
Would it be useful to you to become part of a network of people who are interested in the same topic (regional, national and international)?:

Figure 16.1. Forensic psychiatric questionnaire.

Forensic nursing resource homepage

The National Forensic Nurses' Research and Development Group also discussed the potential advantages of using the Internet as a means of identification of R&D initiatives and dissemination. Use of the Forensic Nursing Resource Homepage (a recent Internet Web innovation by Phil Woods, a nurse academic from the 'family' of forensic nursing) allowed the group to disseminate its activities on an international basis and advertise the database. Persons accessing the resource page to read about the database could also respond. Completed on-screen questionnaires were e-mailed directly to R&D at Rampton Hospital for input into the master database.

The data input at the CRD was carried out in December 1997 using the Idealist database. Each questionnaire was entered directly onto the database, transferring information given by the sender. The description was occasionally edited to enable clarification, keeping the information concise and accurate. Databases such as Idealist are familiar within library searches for information and enable the user to enter key words such as 'author' or 'topic'. In addition to entering the key information outlined in Figure 16.1, additional coding variables to enable other parameters for analysis were input; these included, for example, type of development – whether practice, service or R&D. A regional code and three key search words need to be entered into the database to enable key words to be listed.

Dissemination

Following data input, the CRD carried out final checks to ensure the correct data format before making multicopies of the database in read-only format. Dissemination is based upon the master forensic directory used for the questionnaire distribution, which will ensure that forensic and related units will have access to the information contained within it. In addition, libraries and academic institutions were also targeted with copies. A total of 130 disks containing the database were distributed. Since copyright is not restricted, this also allows users to install the data on more than one computer.

Database content

The database consists of 150 entries within the first dissemination, a remarkable achievement considering that few could be identified within the CRD regional profiling. The national database soon became international with help from the circulation of questionnaires to people working in forensic services abroad and the direct access via the Internet Web page. Countries represented within the database are Australia, Austria, Canada, England, the Netherlands, Norway, Scotland, the USA and Wales.

Multidisciplinary issues

The current drive towards multiprofessional R&D was foremost in thought during the database development: references purely to nursing were avoided wherever possible. Those completing the questionnaire were asked to indicate whether their programmes were multidisciplinary. Figure 16.2 shows that 80% reported developments to include at least two disciplines. Such evidence starts to dispel the myth that multidisciplinary working is relatively undeveloped in R&D. This was further supported by examining the professions' contributions to the database. Programme leaders included nurses (66), psychologists (32), psychiatrists (24), occupational therapists (13), social workers (7) and other professionals such as prison health care workers and probation staff (8). These projects concerned MDOs with enduring mental illnesses, personality disorders and learning disabilities, women's services and prison health care issues in both forensic NHS and non-NHS facilities. The majority of programmes – 75% – fall within the NHS, 19% within private facilities, 5% within universities and 1% within the Ministry of Justice (the Netherlands). Figure 16.3 indicates the number of entries for each forensic service.

Multidisciplinary 80%

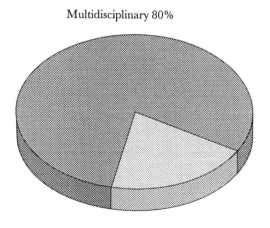

Undisciplinary 20%

Figure 16.2. Multidisciplinary content.

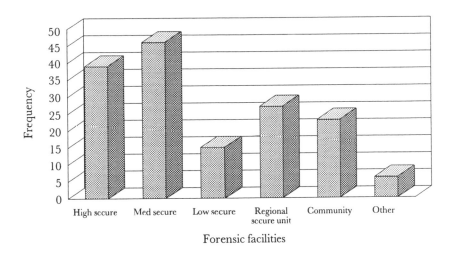

Figure 16.3. Forensic facility representation.

Developing practice

Of the 150 projects registered, only 20% were funded externally to the organisation. This shows the commitment of professionals to developing R&D through personal interest and organisational support. Such programmes also need appropriate resources and academic support. Within the database, 60% of projects were identified as being research based. This does not necessarily mean that these have grown from, or as a result of, direct research but that they may well have drawn upon other research evidence (literature) or elements of the research process. Fifty-five per cent of the programmes directly affected improvements to patient care, 63% affected service developments, and 45% related to outcome measures of the health status of patients.

During the original CRD profiling of the regions, the identification of so few forensic programmes was astonishing despite the knowledge that much work was ongoing. It is sometimes difficult to get people to share their work, and the effort to identify R&D programmes has shown some of the considerable innovations that are occurring. Figure 16.4 identifies the regions that have so far contributed to the forensic database. Originally, the data drew upon the profiling of four regions, with fewer than 20 recorded programmes; at the time of writing 150 programmes are from all NHS regions with international inputs.

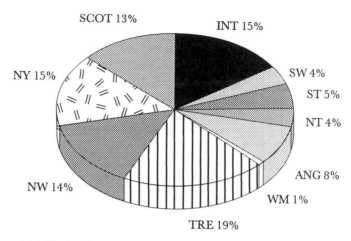

Figure 16.4. Regional representation
Key: INT = International; SW = South West; ST = South Thames; NT = North
Thames; ANG = Anglia and Oxford; WM = West Midlands; TRE - Trent; NW =
North West; NY = Northern and Yorkshire; SCOT = Scotland.

How do people access the database?

First, acquire the disk; then install the database on a personal
computer – it is supplied with easy-to-follow instructions about how
to do this. Then what? Well, it's always good to check out your own
work! If your friends completed a questionnaire, you could always
look them up too. If you do nothing else with it, the database is a
total waste of time. So what could the database be used for? Use your
imagination: how could the data be useful in your work? Focus in on
one clinical area in your practice and think it through using the 150
or more key forensic and related search words to help. Search for a
subject area in which you are interested and use this as a basis to seek
further information. For example, risk assessment is an important
area within forensic health care, and there are over 20 related entries
in the database. If you wanted to develop practice in the area of risk
assessment, there are two ways that the database could help:

- *Time.* The database provides a quick and easy way to see what
  work is under way or has already been completed, which helps to
  stop you 'reinventing the wheel'. In addition, it is useful in bringing together information about isolated units spread across the
  country and informs you of areas of work not being done, which
  is also incredibly valuable.
- *Networking.* The database encourages the sharing of ideas *locally* by
  using the telephone or meeting someone working in a nearby

place, also enabling mutual support to be offered; *regionally*, examining issues via telephoning, seminars or collaborative working; and *nationally*, through seminars, conferences, special interest groups or e-mail discussion forums.

The database does not critique the programmes in any way; instead it provides a resource and catalogue of ongoing forensic-related R&D. With any programme, the user should find out more about it and evaluate its worth against its potential use for the area being considered. The database, if used correctly, offers time-saving and networking in sharing ideas to promote forensic psychiatric innovations. Relevant e-mail and Web addresses appear in the reference section of this chapter.

A model for evidence-based care

Evidence-based practice is a policy imperative highlighted within NHS's R&D strategies (Department of Health, 1991a, 1992b), which indicate that it may be unethical not to practise nursing based upon research. The benefits to patients and health care professionals of basing practice on research findings are becoming more and more recognised and have been reinforced on many occasions (Barnard, 1980; Bergman, 1990; Brown, 1995; Dickoff et al, 1975; Hockey, 1984; Royal College of Nursing, 1982). Despite the acceptance of this principle, the widespread use of evidence on which to base care has yet to be adopted (Jennings and Rodgers, 1988). Evidence-based care involves enabling individuals and organisations to assess, appraise and apply information to everyday situations (Summerton, 1995); it should be seen as a means of enhancing the role of information in decision-making and not an end in itself (Long and Harrison, 1995). Peckham (1995) noted that it allows resources to be used to support interventions of real value. The potential impact of research findings on practice are often limited because there is no formal method of application.

In view of this, a working group examined ways in which to overcome the problem in forensic care and subsequently developed a ward-based distance learning package to assist in developing staff skills (Robinson et al, 1997). Accredited by Sheffield Hallam University, the package has implications for all registered nurses in all nursing contexts.

Recent research (Butterworth, 1996; Redfern, 1996; Robinson, 1995, 1996; Robinson and Reed, 1996) has highlighted deficits in the process of nursing care planning, although the accepted approach to nursing care delivery has developed little since its inception (see the recommendations set out in Hayward's 1986 report). Problems relate to inadequate assessments, global and unrealistic care-planning and low levels of intervention. The nursing process has been seen as little more than a paper exercise, which has led to a poor evaluation of care with a limited influence of research on practice.

There are, however, numerous benefits from using the process of nursing, which have been largely unrecognised and fit well with current legislative and professional requirements (Department of Health, 1989, 1991b, 1993a). These include:

- a research-related approach;
- a more systematic process for the assessment of the patient's condition;
- more relevant care-planning;
- more participation by the patient;
- more effective care delivery.

Using the process of nursing should result in a clearer awareness of intent, a systematic outcome of health status and good-quality care, as well as providing key information for purchasers. Authors of various reports have outlined a number of issues that affect implementation, such as managerial and clinical issues, with educational deficits being the most widely reported (Sheehan, 1991). It was with these issues in mind that there needed to be a bridging of the theory–practice gap that would enable health practitioners to enhance their care delivery skills by using research to inform their practice. A small working group was established to examine and develop ward-based learning in relation to evidence-based care at Rampton Hospital Authority in collaboration with Sheffield Hallam University. An educational evidence-based care programme was developed. The work has implications for forensic and general psychiatric care.

Issues in distance learning

Freeing up time for staff members to participate in educational programmes is a considerable problem. The replacement costs of covering those attending courses are immense. In addition, education has been criticised in that it is often distanced from the practical 'hands-on' care given by health care professionals, resulting in the so-called theory–practice gap. Hopton (1996) argued that mental health nursing educators have failed to respond effectively to the challenge of the theory–practice gap; he suggested that detachment from clinical practice by nurse teachers, together with the low involvement of users in the construction and delivery of the curriculum, has seriously hampered the development of an educational provision that accurately reflects the issues surrounding mental health care.

The evidence-based care package requires that ward-based practitioners centre their learning upon the systematic process of care-planning. It requires that practitioners reflectively utilise and disseminate recently published (researched) approaches to care through their clinical skills in assessing, planning, implementing and evaluating care. They should also be able to perceive deficiencies in the literature that may exist in relation to identified client problems. This ward-based learning approach has several advantages over other methods of educational delivery:

- It adopts the use of the research process in practice.
- It takes the learning process to the learner in a clinical setting.
- It integrates with the learner's existing workload.
- It has greater practical application.
- It allows the learner to develop at his or her own pace.
- It does not require as extensive a resourcing as other methods.
- It is more relevant to the client's needs and actively encourages the client's participation in the learning process.

The ward-based learning programme of evidence-based care may minimise some of the issues raised by Hopton (1996) and others, who have challenged nurse educators to devise new ways of bridging the theory–practice gap. The evidence to emerge from its introduction is that individual learners require differing levels of support in completing it. A system of tutor support for each clinical area allows individual learners to negotiate their own level of support, as well as opening up the possibilities for a number of practitioners. What has emerged is the clear indication that ward-based learning packages are complementary to other forms of education provision and not a substitute for other methods of training delivery.

Rationale for evidence-based care

Evidence-based care is the major issue in health care delivery today. The growing expectations of service commissioners and purchasers mean that providers need increasingly to justify the services they deliver (Robinson et al, 1997). Basing care delivery on research evidence is one means by which to demonstrate services that are dynamic and patient led. Close working relationships between clinical staff and clients are essential if the theory–practice gap is to be closed, individual requirements met and health outcomes maintained and improved .

The use of a systematic approach to the delivery of care through assessment, planning, implementation and evaluation will enable health professionals to provide evidence to support their actions. By using this approach and appropriate research skills, knowledge and care can be considerably enhanced. The main aim of the evidence-based care learning package is therefore to develop skills to enhance professional care activity, which is creatively influenced by research evidence.

Evidence-based care programme workbook content

The workbook takes approximately 48 hours to complete and draws considerably on research activity in order to promote evidence-based care and reduce the theory–practice gap. Implementation has been carried out with good results, showing positive improvements in learning through pre and post measures. Most of the content is considered within the clinical context and should form part of everyday clinical activities. Only a small component is spent examining the literature, although this can be extended.

The workbook consists of 27 activities, with time to reflect at critical stages, and is divided into four main sections:

1. the assessment of patient need;
2. planning evidence-based care based on research;
3. the implementation of evidence-based care;
4. the evaluation of evidence-based care.

Assessment of patient need deals with the systematic collection of information and assessment of the client, these being critical to the formulation of the planned intervention. Without good systematic evidence of baseline functioning, individual needs cannot be identified and subsequently influenced by research evidence.

Following the systematic assessment of individual clients' needs and the prioritisation of interventions, it is then possible to formulate the blueprint for therapeutic intervention. However, rather than continue with current known practices, it is essential to examine these in the light of current research. Thus, once the prioritisation of needs has been completed, the appropriate literature can be reviewed in order to inform the plan of care and related therapeutic intervention. Here opportunities exist to challenge or modify current practice in relation to available evidence.

The implementation section deals with nursing interventions, drawing on the evidence-based plan of care. Identifying the skills required for care intervention and forming relationships with clients are central activities for successful care delivery. Implementing the care plan and recording precise details of interactions and related outcomes are essential to good data collection and subsequent analysis.

The evaluation of clinical interventions with the client – based upon the plan of care and influenced by research evidence – is crucial to determining health outcomes against which measures can be taken. Here, the precise data recorded from interventions are analysed and evaluated to determine the progress of the patient, this process giving valuable insights into health outcomes. Over time, a clear picture emerges of progress or a lack of it.

Research and the Internet

Obtaining information for R&D programmes can be difficult, but new technologies offer exciting challenges that should form part of all research and related activities. 'Surfing', 'browsing' and 'navigating' are now familiar words to those who have accessed the space-age world of the Internet (Robinson, 1997). With the world 'at our fingertips', information relating to almost anything can be accessed, including on-line discussion that traverses cultures world wide.

The rapid growth of information technology and its use as an information source is considerable. One of the latest innovations is that of the Internet. Anyone with a modern personal computer, related software and external telephone line can access information systems on a worldwide basis. Furthermore, you do not need to be a computer whizz-kid to use it! One minute you can be talking to a friend in the USA, the next accessing the latest Department of Health press releases or simply browsing through the World Wide Web (WWW).

What is the Internet?

The Internet is the linkage of many thousands of computers at locations around the world so that each is able to communicate with the others, thus providing access to any Internetted computer. The Internet is not a single entity but a set of resources in the form of millions of files and programmes on tens of thousands of computers. It is these which are accessed for the exchange and sharing of information.

To get on the Internet, host access companies are utilised. Such companies provide many interconnected or networked mainframe computers at a single location. Networking allows computers to share resources and tasks, and therefore operate much faster and more efficiently. Such massive resources are therefore capable of doing things that single computers cannot. By connecting an individual computer to a modem and telephone line, it is possible to access data and run programmes that are the basis for many activities.

A modem is simply a box of electronic wizardry that translates and sends and receives computer information through the telephone lines. As far as the telephone operator is concerned, you are using one telephone line, yet you are, when using the Internet, accessing thousands of other computers world wide. These computers may be at different sites, but each is linked to others by an extended network of telephone lines and other connections.

A computer linked to these types of network is accessible from any site. There are literally millions of worldwide users all contributing to various aspects of the Internet. There are so many facilities available through the Internet that it would take many pages of this book to list all the information. The information exchange and learning opportunities within the Internet are limitless. Because of this, it offers tremendous opportunities to develop worldwide communications on health care issues, sharing and developing local, national and international thinking. So what are the features and resources of this space-age technological miracle that health care staff and researchers can access?

On-line reference materials

On-line reference materials add an important element to the learning process. There are hundreds of libraries and reference sources throughout the world that can be accessed using key words, themes, titles or authors. It is perhaps this facility, more than the others, that has implications for health care learning and acquiring new knowledge. This facility has the ability to bring into the user's home libraries from across the world.

Forums

Creating and participating in electronic forums is one exciting way to acquire knowledge and enhance and contribute to health care practice through creative discussion. Forums are simply groups of people discussing areas of mutual interest and using computers to communicate directly with each other. There are literally thousands of forums discussing all manner of things, and there is already a considerable number of health care forums. For example, there is a forensic discussion group managed from a hospital in Canada that conducts regular discussions on topical issues.

Forums can be visited to find out what worldwide participants have been contributing or asking in relation to specific topics. At specific times, members can talk freely using their keyboard to ask questions and exchange information. One of the most exciting features of participating in electronic forums is the ability to seek and exchange knowledge and views representative of many different cultures. In this environment, the learning situation is on an international basis, people contributing their views and knowledge from many different sources and angles.

Electronic mail

Electronic mail (e-mail) is a way to exchange information, letters, abstracts and reports through electronic channels on a worldwide basis. Documents can be sent to anybody who has a computer and modem facilities and an e-mail/Internet or equivalent identification number. Similarly, the system allows the user to receive new mail. Documents may also be sent to fax machines. Once the host system is running and the telephone line opened, the software automatically displays a list of the mail messages waiting for the user. Here, the 'get new mail' facility allows the user to identify where the mail messages have come from. The messages can be opened, stored on disk or printed off. Existing files, electronic documents and programmes can also be transferred with mail messages as attachments.

World Wide Web

The WWW (or 'Web') is a myriad of 'text' files scattered throughout the Internet network. These consist of pages of text or graphics that contain the information you are accessing. These Web pages have parts highlighted or marked, which enables users to move from one page on one computer to another page on another computer on the Internet – anywhere in the world. For example, it is possible to access a Web page at the World Health Organisation called 'Research in Forensic Psychiatry', which gives abstract details of research projects. An abstract of interest may be accessed by clicking on to it with the 'mouse' (which will probably access data from another part of the Internet), and more information will appear.

The WWW is probably one of the Internet's most exiting features since it allows users to browse at leisure. Here, the exchange of information is considerable. More and more individuals, universities, hospitals, groups, forums and businesses are setting up Web pages to provide information that would take many hours to find in traditional reference libraries.

Because there is a considerable number of WWW pages and sites (and this is expanding every day), there are far too many to list. However, key word or phrase searches allow specific topics to be identified, which will give the user all the addresses in a particular category. Powerful 'search engines' are used to find information. Search engines search thousands of databases at an extremely rapid rate, checking for the information that has been requested. The mouse can be used here to highlight and access specific areas to be visited and viewed. A search using key words 'forensic-psychiatric-nursing' in 1998 revealed 94,427 documents throughout the world, relating to areas such as forensic psychiatric nursing at work, adult and young offenders, psychiatric training schemes, psychiatry and medicine, and research and treatment issues in forensic psychiatry, to name but a few.

Implications for nursing

Acquiring new knowledge by accessing the Internet has limitless potential. The opportunities to expand and reach out into worldwide references, information and cultures is an exciting way in which to learn and enhance patient care. The Internet is a vast resource available at little cost, providing local, national and international information access. Communicating with other cultures, seeing many different viewpoints along the way, allows the sharing of information that cannot be matched elsewhere. The friendly nature and willingness of users to help others to seek solutions and answers to questions now means that there is no excuse for nursing not to be dynamic.

With such opportunities, health care professionals cannot afford to be left behind. Sharing ideas and seeking new information through the Internet offers exhilarating new challenges to nursing and the NHS; service providers need to invest if they are to keep abreast of change and be part of the growing Internet scene. The Forensic Nursing Homepage is an ideal place for the forensic mental health nurse Internet novice to take the first steps.

Forensic nursing on the Internet

The Forensic Nursing Resource Homepage (developed by Phil Woods in 1997) can be found at:

http://wkweb4.cableinet.co.uk/pwoods1/index.html

It aims to be a forum and resource for nurses to obtain links to other Internet sites and to share their ideas or research reports. The front page is, with kind permission, reproduced here (Figure 16.5). It contains:

- links to other Internet sites of forensic and nursing interest;
- information on the Behavioural Status Index (BSI risk programme) and results of empirical studies surrounding this (Woods et al, 1999);
- research reports related to forensic care;
- details of strategies for dealing with aggression in Norway;
- details of forensic discussion lists and training courses available world wide;
- details of the National Forensic Nurses' Research and Development group and its newsletters, and an on-line form to submit a R&D project to the international database;
- bibliographies on risk assessment/patient dangerousness and patient insight.

The site is linked to Internet training programmes available over the network. Further development potential is unlimited.

Forensic nurses are indebted to Phil Woods for creating and maintaining this unsponsored Homepage. There is the facility to announce conferences, upload on-line Powerpoint presentations for clinicians and researchers unable to attend practice development conferences, and download reports and papers. It is generally a place where nurses may share their ideas and interests, make contacts with others, form

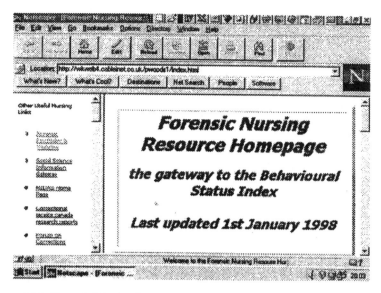

Figure 16.5. Forensic Nursing Resource Homepage

an e-mail link and attach papers or reports. Internet research will be possible via collaborative partnerships forged in this way. Other Internet sites of interest to forensic mental health nurses include:

* http://www.mailbase.ac.uk (health service research)
* http://wwnurse.co./cgi-local/forensic.pl (forensic nursing)
* majordomo@ns.mtroyal.ab.ca (a subscription list for all forensic disciplines at Mount Royal College, Alberta, Canada, accessed via e-mail with the message 'mrcforensiclist')
* listserv@maelstrom.stjohns.edu (a subscription list on forensic psychology and psychiatry, accessed via e-mail using the message 'subscribe forensic-psych')
* listservv@ulkyum.louisville.edu (a subscription list for clinical forensic nursing accessed via e-mail with the message 'subscribe clfornsg')
* listserv@uabdpo.dpouab.edu (a forensic subscription list accessed by e-mail with the message 'subscribe forensic')
* drobin@rampton-hospital.btinternet.com (for more information on the International Forensic Psychiatric Database or the National Forensic Nurses' Research and Development Group)

Conclusions

There are no conclusions to this chapter – just lots of new beginnings.

References

Barnard KE (1980) Knowledge for practice: directions for the future. Nursing Research, 28, 208–12.

Bergman R (1990) Priorities in nursing research: change and continuity. In Bergman R (Ed) Nursing Research for Nursing and Practice. London: Chapman and Hall.

Brooks N (1988) Why research? British Journal of Occupational Therapy 51: 11.

Brown GD (1995) Understanding barriers to basing nursing practice upon research: a communication model approach. Journal of Advanced Nursing 21(1): 154–7.

Butterworth T (1994) Working in Partnership: A Collaborative Approach to Care. London: HMSO.

Butterworth T (1996) Individualised nursing care: a cuckoo in the team's nest? NT Research 1(1): 34–7.

Clark JM, Hockey L (1979) Research for Nursing. Aylesbury: HM&M.

Darling VH, Rodgers I (1986) Research for Practising Nurses. London: Macmillan.

Department of Health (1990) Working for Patients. London: HMSO.

Department of Health (1991a) A Research and Development Strategy for the NHS. London: HMSO.

Department of Health (1991b) The Patient's Charter. London: HMSO.

Department of Health (1992a) Ministerial Review: Draft Action Plan for 1992–3 (7th revision). London: Department of Health.

Department of Health (1992b) The Health of the Nation. London: Department of Health.

Department of Health (1993a) A Vision for the Future: The Nursing and Health Visiting Contribution to Health Care. London: Department of Health/NHS Management Executive.

Department of Health (1993b) Report of the Taskforce on the Strategy for Research in Nursing, Midwifery and Health Visiting. London: HMSO.

Department of Health and Special Hospitals Service Authority (1995) Making the Vision a Reality: Progress Towards Achievement of the Targets Set in 'A Vision for the Future'. London: Department of Health/Special Hospitals Service Authority.

Dickoff J, James P and Semradek J (1975) Eight for research. Part 1: a stance for nursing research – tenacity or enquiry? Nursing Research, 24, 84–8.

Grubin D, Gunn J (1991) Report on a Register of Research Relating to the Mentally Disordered Offender. London: Mental Health Foundation.

Hayward IC (1986) Report of the Nursing Process Evaluation Workshop Group. London: Kings College, University of London.

Heber L (1987) Nursing diagnosis in professional psychiatric nursing. In Hannah K et al (Eds) Clinical Judgement and Decision Making. New York: John Wiley & Sons.

Hockey L (1984) The nature and purpose of research. In Cormack D (Ed.) The Research Process in Nursing. Oxford: Blackwell Scientific Publications.

Hopton J (1996) Reconceptualising the theory–practice gap in mental health nursing. Nurse Education Today 16(3): 227–32.

Jennings BM, Rodgers S (1988) Merging nursing research and practice: a case of multiple identities. Journal of Advanced Nursing 13(6): 752–8.

Long A, Harrison S (1995) The balance of evidence. Health Service Journal: Health Management Guide p 1.

Marsland D (1993) Research and destroy. Nursing Standard 7(32): 45.

Mogg K, Mathews A, Weinman J (1987) Memory bias in clinical anxiety. Journal of Abnormal Psychology 96: 94–8.

Peckham M (1995) The new world of R & D: the challenge for NHS Boards. Health

Director (Nov).

Rae MA (1994) Freedom To Care. Merseyside: Graphics Department, Ashworth Hospital.

Redfern S (1996) Individualised patient care: its meaning and practice in a general setting. NT Research 1(1): 22–33.

Reed J (1992) Review of Health and Social Services for Mentally Disordered Offenders and Others Requiring Similar Services – Final Summary Report. Appendix 1: Advisory Group on Setting Priorities for Mental Health Research and Development. London: HMSO.

Reed V, Dean A (1986) At the theory–practice interface: an inquiry into the facilitation of practitioner research. Proceedings of the International Nursing Research Conference, Edmonton, Alberta, 7–9 May.

Reed V, Robinson DK (1992) The Rampton Hospital Community Liaison Nursing Service: Achievements and Opportunities. London: Special Hospitals Service Authority.

Roberson MHB (1992) The meaning of compliance: patient perspectives. Qualitative Health Research 2(1): 7–26.

Robinson DK (1995) Are nurses fulfilling their proper role?: measuring culture trends in mental health nursing care. Psychiatric Care 2(1): 27–31.

Robinson DK (1996) Measuring psychiatric nursing interactions: how much individualised care? NT Research 1(1): 13–21.

Robinson D (1997) Surfing the Internet: challenges for health care. Psychiatric Care 4(3): 124–6.

Robinson DK, Reed V (1996) Measuring Forensic Psychiatric and Mental Health Nursing Interactions. Aylesbury: Avebury.

Robinson DK, Reed V (1998) A to Z of Social Research Jargon. Aylesbury: Avebury.

Robinson D, Gajos M, Whyte L (1997) Integrating research into practice: a model for evidence based care through ward based learning. Psychiatric Care 4(6): 274–8.

Royal College of Nursing (1982) Research Mindedness and Education. London: RCN.

Sheehan J (1986) Nursing research in Britain: the state of the art. Nurse Education Today 6(1): 3–9.

Sheehan J (1991) Conceptions of the nursing process amongst nurse teachers and clinical nurses. Journal of Advanced Nursing 16(3): 333–42.

Smith JP (1986) The beginning of the end. Senior Nurse 5(1): 14–15.

Special Hospitals Service Authority (1993a) Evaluation of the Impact of Ward Managers in their First Year of Appointment. London: Special Hospitals Service Authority.

Special Hospitals Service Authority (1993b) 'Big, Black and Dangerous'. Report of the Committee of Inquiry into the Death in Broadmoor Hospital of Orville Blackwood and a Review of the Deaths of two Other Afro-Caribbean Patients. London: Special Hospitals Service Authority.

Summerton N (1995) The burden of proof. Health Service Journal (Nov 30): 33.

Taylor P (1991) Research Strategy for the Special Hospitals. London: Special Hospitals Service Authority.

UKCC (United Kingdom Central Council for Nursing, Midwifery and Health Visiting) (1993) Code of Professional Conduct, 3rd Edn. London: UKCC.

Webb C, Mackenzie J (1993) Where are we now?: research mindedness in the 1990s. Journal of Clinical Nursing 2: 129–33.

Woods P, Reed V and Robinson D (1999) The Behavioural Status Index: therapeutic assessment of risk, insight, communication and social skills. Journal of Psychiatric and Mental Health Nursing, 6, 79–80.

Chapter 17
The reliability of predictions of dangerousness: implications for nursing

CHRIS SKELLY

Forensic mental health nurses provide care for a client group whose unifying characteristic is that they have been described as dangerous, a label that will influence the treatment setting, the attitude of the nurse towards the patient and the length of detention. The emphasis on dangerousness as a central concept for this occupational group is perhaps necessary for the process of role identification and delimitation but can be overemphasised, and hence overpredicted, to the detriment of the patient, who may be nursed under greater restrictions than are necessary.

Medical expertise is often assumed in the prediction of dangerousness, this concept being utilised in hospital admission and discharge decisions. Whilst the necessity of involuntary hospitalisation may be evident at the time of admission, at some point subsequent to this the patient may no longer be dangerous but is predicted to remain so and is not discharged. Given the serious consequences of these decisions for compulsorily detained mentally disordered patients, it is important that nurses re-examine their assumptions about dangerousness and establish an autonomous role, in terms of its prediction, that more correctly addresses the concerns for nursing.

Dangerousness

Dangerousness is a subjective concept for which many definitions have been formulated. The intention here is not to add another to the list but briefly to explicate some practical effects of existing definitions. No one definition may be universally acceptable, but a knowl-

edge of several can contribute to a better understanding and opera-
tionalisation of the concept.

A useful place to start is with the view proposed by the Committee on Mentally Abnormal Offenders that dangerousness is 'a
propensity to cause serious physical injury or lasting psychological
harm' (Home Office and Department of Health and Social Security,
1975). This is a commonly accepted view that, for all its relative
simplicity, has value in introducing the issue of psychological harm.
This is a contentious aspect as psychological harm may arise from
non-violent acts, and individual susceptibility to such harm may be a
factor related to the victim rather than the harmful behaviour. The
effect of this is to extend the range of those behaviours and those
individuals considered to be dangerous beyond that of less inclusive
definitions.

In a forensic nursing context, Tarbuck (1994) has suggested that
dangerousness is 'the probability that an individual will commit a
violent act upon the person of another (or others) in the near or
distant future, if afforded the opportunity to do so'. Whilst this does
not identify the severity or the nature of the harm inflicted, it does
raise the issue of opportunity. In a secure setting, the opportunities
for dangerous behaviour are restricted by treatment, physical control
and isolation from potential victims. The absence of dangerous
behaviour in a detained patient may consequently be due to a lack of
opportunity rather than a reduction of dangerous tendencies, which
presents difficulties when discharge decisions are based primarily
upon an assessment of behaviour in hospital.

A third definition that could be considered is that of Scott (1977),
who defined dangerousness as 'an unpredictable and untreatable
tendency to inflict or risk serious, irreversible injury or destruction,
or to induce others to do so'. This suggests that, if the behaviour
could be predicted and treated, it would no longer be dangerous. To
the extent that patients detained in hospital are predicted to be
dangerous and their condition is considered to be treatable, this can,
at first sight, lead to the counterintuitive conclusion that, by this definition, such patients are not dangerous. This conclusion, in fact,
often proves to be true – that, in a secure setting, most detained
patients are not dangerous for most of the time (possibly because of
the lack of opportunity) and that the patients who are dangerous
within the secure setting are those who remain either unpredictable
or untreatable.

The relationship between dangerousness and mental illness

The mentally ill are commonly stereotyped by the public as being more prone to violence than the rest of society (Mullen, 1984; Rabkin, 1974). This perception has been reinforced in recent years by the media coverage of a number of serious assaults and homicides committed by psychiatric patients in the community, a situation that may indicate not the inherent dangerousness of psychiatric patients but inadequacies in discharge and aftercare provision.

Many researchers have found little evidence to endorse the supposition that mental illness increases the risk of violence (Hafner and Boker,1982; Teplin, 1985), although there may be subgroups among the mentally abnormal who have higher rates of conviction for violent behaviour that predates their hospitalisation (Steadman et al, 1978). These subgroups are generally those described as suffering from psychopathy, alcoholism and drug addiction rather than those with a mental illness (Guze, 1976). Where studies have found a relationship, this appears to be as a result of active symptoms of psychosis (Junginger, 1996) rather than a history of mental illness (Mulvey, 1994).

The relationship between dangerousness and mental illness is considered by Szasz (1963) to be mythical, being formed in part by the ascription of mental illness to those individuals who have engaged in dangerous behaviour. The relationship may, however, be factual for psychiatric inpatients, especially those who are compulsorily detained. This should not be altogether unexpected given that the principal justification for compulsorily detained is dangerousness. Although several studies have noted the association of hospitalisation with pre- and post-admission violence (for example, Lagos et al, 1977; McNiel and Binder, 1989), Steadman (1981), in contrast, maintains that there is no evidence of any direct relationship between assaultive behaviour in mental hospitals and in the community as violence may be situationally determined. This may not be true for acutely ill people in the community who are admitted involuntarily to hospital but has some credence when considering the discharge of the patient back to the community: that violence displayed in the hospital may not be the result of mental illness but of the frustrations of institutional existence, and may not be evidence of continuing dangerousness and unsuitability for discharge.

Prediction: actuarial, clinical ... or political?

Actuarial methods of prediction aim to differentiate the dangerous from the non-dangerous by isolating the relevant factors from an examination of the demographic variables of those who have previously exhibited dangerous behaviour. Cocozza and Steadman (1974) developed a Legal Dangerousness Scale (LDS), which they applied retrospectively to the 'Baxstrom' cohort. This was a group of 967 detained patients who were considered to be dangerous by medical staff but were transferred to non-secure hospitals as the result of a US Supreme Court decision in 1966. The LDS took into account the arrest and conviction history as well as the severity of the original offence. Although the LDS in combination with age could accurately identify the dangerous patients, as these represented fewer than a third of all patients so identified, it provided inadequate criteria for differentiating them from the non-dangerous patients.

Research studies are unanimous that the best predictor of violent crime is a previous conviction for it and that each conviction increases the probability of a further conviction (Craft, 1984). By the time of the third conviction, the probability of a further conviction is 60% (Walker, 1982). Aside from offence patterns, most demographic variables cannot be used to predict outcomes (Sepejak et al, 1983), although a number of factors have been found to be closely related to violence; these include age, sex, race, socio-economic status and opiate/alcohol abuse – but not mental illness in the absence of a history of violence (Monahan, 1981). Actuarial methods can prove useful in predicting the probability of dangerous behaviour within a large group, but they are less useful for identifying the individual within the group who is dangerous; for this, clinical methods are more appropriate.

Clinicians have emphasised a number of different traits as being of significance in assessing dangerousness, for example the ability to feel compassion for others and to learn by experience (Scott, 1977), temper tantrums in an adult, a vengeful attitude and a facility with weapons (Loucas, 1982). However, even if these dispositional traits were correlated with dangerousness, it is not apparent whether they occur with any greater frequency than in the non-dangerous. Such an approach of individual psychopathology stems from the medical model, which then directs research to find more accurate dispositional measures that will differentiate the dangerous from the non-dangerous.

These traits in isolation do not fully account for dangerousness, which may more conceivably be a potential reaction that is triggered by particular situations (Home Office and Department of Health and Social Security, 1975). Megargee (1976) proposes a model in which motivation, internal inhibition and habit strength are important factors, along with situational circumstances such as environmental stress, the availability of a weapon and the presence of a potential victim. This emphasis on environmental factors poses a further problem when making a prediction of dangerousness: if it is difficult to predict from the individual's enduring, and known, characteristics, it may be even more difficult to predict from the varied, and unknown, situations that an individual will encounter in the future.

In a comparison between clinical and actuarial studies, Sawyer (1966) concluded that actuarial methods were the more accurate. However, as predictions of violence amongst the mentally disordered are wrong at least twice as often as they are correct (Monahan, 1984), and the accuracy of prediction, even among extremely high-risk groups, rarely exceeds that of chance, the best strategy is still to predict non-violence, all other types of predictions increasing the error rate by identifying false positives (Steadman, 1983). The transfer of the 'Baxstrom' patients enabled an assessment to be made of the proportion of false positives (those wrongly predicted to be dangerous) in a population considered to be dangerous. At a 1-year follow-up, only 7 (out of 967) were back in a secure setting, giving a rate of 137 false positives for every false negative (those wrongly predicted to be safe). A similar group of 586 mentally ill offenders, transferred in similar circumstances from a hospital in Pennsylvania in 1971, were similarly found not to be as dangerous as predicted: at a 4-year follow-up, only 14.5% could be classified as dangerous (Thornberry and Jacoby, 1979). It is unclear, however, just how 'dangerous' these groups of patients actually were and whether they could be considered as constituting a population comparable to those who are detained in secure institutions in this country. In this context it is interesting to note that it has been estimated that 35–50% of patients in high security hospitals (for England and Wales) do not require this level of security (Maden et al., 1995).

The inaccurate overprediction of dangerousness inevitably leads to some safe people being detained in secure hospitals. These false positives are difficult to detect as their lack of dangerous behaviour is attributed to the benefits of treatment and their continued detention denies them the opportunity to disprove the prediction. Conversely, those who behave violently while in hospital confirm the prediction even though the violence may be caused by unique situational factors. Any normal behaviour, or behaviour that is normal in a closed institution, can be interpreted to validate the correctness of a prediction (Rosenhan, 1973), and being treated as dangerous can be a self-fulfilling prophecy in that the patient responds violently to the way in which he is being treated. As the false positives are not easily identified within the hospital, their situation attracts little attention, greater public, professional and political concern being shown over the false negatives who offend after discharge and have a disproportionate effect on mental health policy. The belief that psychiatric patients are dangerous is maintained by this bias of concern (Crawford, 1984), resulting in the dilemma for involuntary hospitalisation:

> how many probably safe individuals should cautious policy continue to detain in hospitals in the hope of preventing the release of one who is still potentially dangerous? (Home Office and Department of Health and Social Security, 1975)

The unfortunate truth is that many may be unnecessarily detained as those responsible for discharge decisions are likely to err on the side of caution, a practice identified by Thornberry and Jacoby (1979) as 'political prediction'. By perpetuating the detention, criticism is avoided as the prediction is never put to the test.

The role of the psychiatrist

Psychiatrists have been accorded the role of expert in the prediction of future violent behaviour amongst the mentally ill without ever having offered any evidence of such expertise, research in fact presenting convincing evidence that they have no such special expertise (Cocozza and Steadman, 1976). Psychiatry's involvement follows from its role in the diagnosis and treatment of mental illness and the perceived association of mental illness with dangerous behaviour. Again, research fails to confirm the underlying assumptions: that mental illness can be reliably diagnosed, that it is related to dangerousness and that predictions of dangerousness are accurate and reliable (Crawford, 1984).

The ability of psychiatrists to predict dangerousness in a group of mentally ill offenders has been demonstrated to be no better than that of teachers (Quinsey and Ambtman, 1979). The psychiatrists were also found not to employ any specialised assessment techniques in arriving at their judgements. Montandon and Harding (1984) similarly found no higher level of agreement between psychiatrists than between non-psychiatrists, and the psychiatrists generally gave the highest ratings of dangerousness even for cases with no indication of mental illness or violence. The evidence suggests that psychiatrists base their judgements on non-medical information that others are at least as competent to interpret (Bowden, 1985).

The dissonance between the assumptions and the reality has led to the accusation that 'the emperor has no clothes' (Steadman, 1983), but in fairness it should be noted that psychiatrists are expected to judge on the dangerous/not dangerous dichotomy rather than indicating a position on a continuum of probability. In the absence of any valid predictors of dangerousness, it has been suggested that their primary task should be not that of accurate prediction but that of explanation of the clinical decision-making process and of how defensible the prediction is (Pollock et al, 1989).

The role of the nurse

In studying the role of the forensic mental health nurse, it was found that 84% of those surveyed felt that they should have knowledge of assessing dangerousness (Kitchiner et al, 1992). But should nursing be just one more discipline that makes inaccurate assessments and predictions of dangerousness when we know that such actions often work to the detriment of the patient? Mental health nurses are in a position to select and control the flow of information concerning the patient, and are thus, as Fischer (1989) notes, able to interfere with the patient's liberty. Nurses must recognise their responsibility to the patient in ensuring the accuracy of information gained in their relationship with the patient. Unfortunately, these are issues that can easily take second place to the social control function of the nurse, a role itself legitimated in the *Code of Professional Conduct* by placing a responsibility on the nurse to serve the interests of society (UKCC, 1992).

The traditional role of the nurse, when involved in assessing and predicting dangerousness, is to elicit information concerning the patient from observation and verbal interaction and to share this with the multidisciplinary clinical team. Despite the limitations of the ward environment, useful information can be gained, including some estimation of the patient's dispositional traits, response to stressful situations, available coping mechanisms, problem-solving

skills, development towards more appropriate interpersonal relationships and progress through incremental steps of controlled risk-
taking. Violent incidents themselves need not be viewed wholly
negatively as they can provide a learning experience, for both the
nurse and the patient, of the causes of violence and how the patient
can best learn to control his violent impulses.

Within an institutional setting, three particular problems may
beset nursing staff in their consideration of dangerousness, which
can result in its overprediction. First, an empirical association may
be formed between mental illness and dangerousness because of
positive selection for just these characteristics in those admitted.
Second, in the absence of knowledge of the true predictors, dangerousness may be simply inferred from the institutional surroundings.
The patient admitted to a secure institution may initially be labelled
as dangerous as a result of his behaviour but may subsequently be so
labelled because he is in a secure institution. Third, an area often
exclusively undertaken by nursing staff is the prediction, prevention
and management of imminent violence. Here, the nurse may
attribute excessive import to inpatient violence as a predictor of
future dangerousness as nurses are often the victims or have to deal
with its consequences.

Developing a theoretical framework

Nurses in secure settings utilise a range of nursing models without
any consensus on which is the more appropriate for this particular
client group. Few of the published models have been developed
specifically for the psychiatric patient and none for the dangerous
psychiatric patient. The 'dangerous' nature of the patient may be
overridden by other concerns, such as his need for self-care skills or
psychodynamic interventions, which may direct the choice of a nursing model. The appropriateness of these models has to be tested in
secure settings as some needs may not be met as a result of environmental constraints rather than the patient's behaviour. It may be
Utopian to expect a specific forensic model to be developed, but a
'best fit' model is needed that provides a better theoretical framework than the medical model for assessing dangerousness, that
emphasises the situational determinants of dangerous behaviour and
that takes into account the patient's responsibility to society. Nursing
models have, however, failed to deliver in this area.

Whilst some secure settings use systematic methods for assessing dangerousness and risk, these often function as checklists rather than as predictive instruments. Their utility is in ensuring that all relevant factors are considered in assessing the patient and as an aid to where to direct treatment to ameliorate the risk. It remains uncertain whether these methods improve outcomes and whether a systematic, but atheoretical, process has advantages over a more intuitive method. Whichever method of assessment and prediction is employed, there is a need for longitudinal study to evaluate the predictions made for each individual, such feedback having the power to educate and to alter assumptions.

Advocacy

In recent years, the role of the nurse as an advocate for the patient has gained prominence. In a bureaucratised health service, the patient is in a relatively powerless position, this then being exacerbated by mental illness, which can further reduce the patient's ability to participate actively in his treatment. The consequences of compulsory detention are severe, which adds further impetus to the need for a proactive advocate. Although the need is there, some argue that nurses are not suited to this role because of their part in the health structure and their role as agents of social control (McFadyen, 1989; Porter, 1988). Advocacy is another – and potentially conflicting – role recognised in the *Code of Professional Conduct* (UKCC, 1992) in emphasising the safeguarding of the interests of individual patients.

To act as an advocate, the nurse must engage in an open and honest relationship with the patient, who must be kept informed of progress and actively involved in his treatment plan. This co-operative approach can of itself do much to redress the adversarial nature of the nurse–patient relationship in some secure settings. The nurse can act as patient advocate in a number of specific ways, including advising the patient of his legal rights concerning medication and discharge through proposing increased stages of liberty for the patient via informed risk taking. Unsubstantiated assertions of dangerousness can be counteracted by examining the evidence and weighing this against the patient's capacity for non-dangerous behaviour obtained via a comprehensive nursing assessment. The interpretation of behaviours as pathological should not go unchallenged either, and the patient should be encouraged to access his clinical records to validate the interpretations given or to enable alternative explanations to be offered. The aim should be to ensure that decisions concerning the patients liberty are based on accurate information rather than assumption.

Conclusions

None of the foregoing discussion is meant to suggest that all detained psychiatric patients are unjustly detained: many would be highly dangerous within the community. For the benefit of society, it is necessary to try to identify these patients, particularly within populations that have a high base rate for this behaviour. Unfortunately, it is difficult accurately to segregate the dangerous from the non-dangerous amongst the hospital population, with the result that dangerousness is assumed on the Utilitarian principle of the requirements of public safety dominating the potential (and lesser) harm to the individual patient.

The aim of this chapter has been to put the assessment and prediction of dangerousness into its proper perspective. The nurse needs to be aware that the continued dangerousness of patients is often directly related to their having previously committed a dangerous act rather than to the presence of mental illness. The equivocal nature of the relationship between mental illness and dangerousness, the unreliability of its prediction and the harmful effects for many patients have all been identified. Alerted by this knowledge, there are two tasks before the nurse. First, the nurse should continue the search for more accurate predictors by the development and testing of risk assessment formats. Second, in the present 'state of the art', the nurse should act as advocate for the patient and not collude with others in making innaccurate predictions based upon false premiss.

References

Bowden P (1985) Psychiatry and dangerousness: a counter renaissance? In Gostin L (Ed.) Secure Provision. London: Tavistock.

Cocozza JJ, Steadman HJ (1974) Some refinements in the measurement and prediction of dangerous behaviour. American Journal of Psychiatry 131(9): 1012–14.

Cocozza JJ, Steadman HJ (1976) The failure of psychiatric predictions of dangerousness: clear and convincing evidence. Rutgers Law Review 29: 1084–101.

Craft M (1984) Predicting dangerousness and future convictions among the mentally abnormal. In Craft M, Craft A (Eds) Mentally Abnormal Offenders. London: Baillière Tindall.

Crawford D (1984) Problems with the assessment of dangerousness in England and Wales. Medicine and Law 3: 141–50.

Fischer A (1989) The Process of Definition and Action: The Case of Dangerousness. California: University of California.

Guze S (1976) Criminality and Psychiatric Disorders. New York: Oxford University Press.

Hafner H, Boker W (1982) Crimes of Violence by Mentally Abnormal Offenders. Cambridge: Cambridge University Press.

Home Office and Department of Health and Social Security (1975) Report of the Committee on Mentally Abnormal Offenders. London: HMSO.

Junginger J (1996) Psychosis and violence: the case for a context analysis of psychotic experience. Schizophrenia Bulletin 22(1): 91–103.

Kitchiner N, Wright I, Topping-Morris B, Burnard P, Morrison P (1992) The role of the forensic psychiatric nurse. Nursing Times 88(8): 56.

Lagos J, Perlmutter K, Saexinger H (1977) Fear of the mentally ill: empirical support for the common man's response. American Journal of Psychiatry 134: 1134–7.

Loucas K (1982) Assessing dangerousness in psychotics. In Hamilton J, Freeman H (Eds) Dangerousness: Psychiatric Assessment and Management. London: Gaskell.

Maden A, Curle C, Meux C, Burrow S, Gunn J (1995) Treatment and Security Needs of Special Hospital Patients. London: Whurr.

McFadyen JA (1989) Who will speak for me? Nursing Times 85(6): 45–8.

McNiel D, Binder R (1989) Relationship between preadmission threats and later violent behaviour by acute psychiatric in-patients. Hospital and Community Psychiatry 40(6): 605–8.

Megargee EI 1976) The prediction of dangerous behaviour. Criminal Justice and Behaviour 3(1): 3–22.

Monahan J (1981) Predicting Violent Behaviour: An Assessment of Clinical Techniques. Beverley Hills: Sage.

Monahan J (1984) The prediction of violent behaviour: toward a second generation of theory and policy. American Journal of Psychiatry 141(1): 1–15.

Montandon C, Harding T (1984) The reliability of dangerousness assessments: a decision making exercise. British Journal of Psychiatry 144: 149–55.

Mullen P (1984) Mental disorder and dangerousness. Australian and New Zealand Journal of Psychiatry 18: 8–17.

Mulvey E (1994) Assessing the evidence of a link between mental illness and violence. Hospital and Community Psychiatry 45(7): 663–8.

Pollock N, McBain I, Webster C (1989) Clinical decision making and the assessment of dangerousness. In Howells K, Hollin C (Eds) Clinical Approaches to Violence. Chichester: John Wiley & Sons.

Porter S (1988) Siding with the system. Nursing Times 84(41): 3–31.

Quinsey V, Ambtman R (1979) Variables affecting psychiatrists' and teachers' assessments of the dangerousness of mentally ill offenders. Journal of Consulting and Clinical Psychology 47(2): 353–62.

Rabkin J (1974) Attitudes towards mental illness. Schizophrenia Bulletin 10: 7–33.

Rosenhan D (1973) On being sane in insane places. Science 179: 25-28.

Sawyer J (1966) Measurement and prediction, clinical and statistical. Psychological Bulletin 66: 178–200.

Scott P (1977) Assessing dangerousness in criminals. British Journal of Psychiatry 131: 127–42.

Sepejak D, Menzies R, Webster C, Jensen F (1983) Clinical predictions of dangerousness: two-year follow-up of 408 pre-trial forensic cases. Bulletin of the American Academy of Psychiatry and the Law 11(2): 171–81.

Steadman H (1981) Special problems in the prediction of violence among the mentally ill. In Hays T, Roberts T, Solway K (Eds) Violence and the Violent Individual. New York: Spectrum.

Steadman H (1983) Predicting dangerousness among the mentally ill: art, magic and science. International Journal of Law and Psychiatry 6: 381–90.

Steadman H, Cocozza J, Melick M (1978) Explaining the increased arrest rate among mental patients: the changing clientele of state hospitals. American Journal of Psychiatry 135: 816–820.

Szasz T (1963) Law, Liberty and Psychiatry. New York: Macmillan.

Tarbuck P (1994) The therapeutic use of security: a model for forensic nursing. In Thompson T, Mathias P (Eds) Lyttle's Mental Health and Disorder, 2nd Edn. London: Baillière Tindall.

Teplin L (1985) The criminality of the mentally ill: a dangerous misconception. American Journal of Psychiatry 142(5): 593–9.

Thornberry T, Jacoby J (1979) The Criminally Insane: A Community Follow-up of Mentally Ill Offenders. Chicago: University of Chicago Press.

UKCC (United Kingdom Central Council for Nursing, Midwifery and Health Visiting) (1992) Code of Professional Conduct, 3rd Edn. London: UKCC.

Walker N (1982) Ethical aspects of detaining dangerous people. In Hamilton J, Freeman H (Eds) Dangerousness: Psychiatric Assessment and Management. London: Gaskell.

Chapter 18
Care and responsibility training: survey of skills retention and diminution

PAUL TARBUCK, YVONNE EATON, JOE McAULIFFE, MICK RUANE and BILL THORPE

Different opinions are held on the frequency and nature of the periodic refreshment of the skills associated with care and responsibility training (formerly control and restraint training), colloquially known as C&R. Received wisdom imparted to the teachers of C&R from the original instructors of C&R (at the Home Office) suggested that – after receiving the initial period of instruction (a minimum of 5 days and more usually 10) – students would require updating on an annual basis, and if the student did not attend within 12 months, a whole foundation course should be re-taken.

At Ashworth Hospital, every member of the nursing workforce between 1993 and 1996 was facilitated to study C&R techniques and associated topics for at least 2 days per annum (Dale et al, 1995; Tarbuck, 1994). The writers decided that the original proposition concerning the frequency of C&R updating should be tested and that an assessment of C&R skills retention and diminution would assist with the development of the curriculum.

Ashworth Hospital

Ashworth Hospital Authority is an NHS high-security facility, one of three, serving the populations of England and Wales. Ashworth is situated on Merseyside, 12 miles from the conurbation of Liverpool. It has a campus of 42 acres on two sites, some 500 beds and a multidisciplinary staff complement of approximately 1500. Ashworth was formerly known as a 'Special Hospital', and its admission criteria are centred upon the prospective patient being 'a grave and immediate

229

risk' to the public and also on the premise that the individual has a treatable disorder.

The literature

No literature concerning skill retention and diminution within C&R training is available, although a number of articles concerning general principles associated with the use of C&R techniques exist and are pertinent to this discussion. The position statements of the Royal College of Nursing (Bates et al, 1997; Royal College of Nursing, 1992) indicate that it is good practice for education and training in the management of violent incidents to be made available to all staff who care for individuals with these propensities. It is critical to note that training encompasses a range of interventions for assaultive persons only the last of which, when all others have been exhausted without success, should be of a physically controlling nature. The extent of training should be determined by local need and in the context of individual performance review.

Aiken and Tarbuck (1995) discussed the ethical and legal bases of care of the assaultive individual and proposed a framework to guide practice (Epsilon Publishers, 1994), Kidd and Stark (1995) published a guide to care of the aggressive individual, and Tarbuck (1992a, 1992b) indicated that, in units where nurses utilise verbal and interpersonal skills to good effect, managers should be aware that physical methods of control are likely to be used infrequently and that employees may become deskilled as they do not practise C&R techniques regularly. Paradoxically, this phenomenon is most welcome as non-invasive interventions are always preferable to physical ones. However, in these circumstances, the regular updating of staff in C&R techniques is desirable, although such a programme may have significant resourcing implications for employing authorities.

A teaching maxim suggests that skills are more completely assimilated into the repertoire of behaviours of students when they not only have had the skill modelled to them, but also have had the opportunity to practise the skill. This suggests that a person without the opportunity to practise a skill may not completely assimilate the skill and is potentially susceptible to the corruption of the skill. There is long experience concerning the acquisition of first aid training skills, which suggests that skills should be updated every 3 years with regard to basic techniques and that the more advanced techniques require annual updating (St John Ambulance, 1992). Trainers at Ashworth Hospital, who teach both C&R and first aid skills, had suggested that the principles underpinning the two courses (cognitive and psychomotor) are not too dissimilar and that periodic updating would be the optimum model for C&R, as it is for first aid skills training. The recommendation of C&R update training occurring on an annual basis was contentious as it was based on 'received wisdom' rather than evidence.

Parkes (1996) studied the effectiveness of control and restraint training in a medium secure unit. He noted an increase in staff injury during incidents involving those who had received training (he did not indicate the level of injury to the persons subject to restraint, which would have been interesting). Parkes attributed the increased injury rate to teams using C&R approaching from the front of (rather than from behind) an assaultive person. However, Stansfield (1998) has demonstrated an increase in confidence in the staff members so trained. Could it be that the restraint teams may have been overconfident of their ability to control a person and, once committed, had to wrestle with him or her rather more than had been anticipated?

Care and responsibility training

C&R training was recommended by the Ritchie Report (1984) for introduction into the Special Hospitals, and it has subsequently cascaded into the medium secure sector and mainstream NHS. C&R was created by the Physical Education branch of Her Majesty's Prison Service and comprises a number of systematic techniques that may be employed to assist one to break away from being held against one's wishes, and to control an assaultive individual using a three-person team. A further specialist derivation is also available concerning the use of protective equipment. C&R training has now been subjected to educational principles, and insights into training are available in video-assisted Open Learning packages (Epsilon Publishers, 1994).

C&R has matured within the NHS and is now substantially different from the original Home Office/prison service provision in that a therapeutic value system has been introduced that is concerned with returning autonomy and control to the individual rather than with the simple and efficient control of individuals with 'assaultive' behaviours. The Royal College of Nursing (1994) has published a syllabus of training for instructors of control and restraint. Ashworth Hospital has led this change in emphasis and has adopted the nomenclature of 'care and responsibility' (in preference to control and restraint) to reflect this crucial and fundamental ideological shift. New variants of C&R training have proliferated over the past decade, and, without a centralised regulatory system, there is room for a wide array of 'orthodoxy'. The problem of aggression and violence in the NHS workplace is now so common that most large NHS provider services employ their own retain C&R trainers on the staff. Some specialised forms of training are also available for deployment by staff members caring for the older adult or young persons.

Method

The C&R training department, having decided to undertake this survey, agreed to create a video recording of 10 essential C&R techniques (Table 18.1). This videotape record of 'orthodox' practice was to be used to provide a visual control against which all C&R techniques would be adjudged for competency. A form was developed upon which recordings would be made concerning students' previous exposure to C&R training, skills diminution and retention, on entry to and after update instruction. This form tabulated the 10 essential techniques and allowed spaces for marks and comments to be inserted. Each course participant was evaluated concurrently by two teachers of C&R, who recorded their impressions of the student using the survey tool; reference was made to the video recording if a comparator was needed to check the orthodoxy of a technique. The survey took 3 months to complete.

Table 18.1. Ten essential care and responsibility techniques

Technique	Description
1	Principles of a wrist hold
2	Principles of a straight arm hold
3	Securing the head and airway
4	Transfer of hold – standing
5	Transfer of hold – front
6	Transfer of hold – back
7	Removal of hands from object
8	Front stranglehold – release
9	Rear stranglehold – release
10	Hair grabs

The participants comprised 18 personnel from Ashworth and 28 NHS personnel, giving a sample group of 46 students (n = 46). All the students had completed an initial C&R course and were now undertaking C&R updating within:

- 12 months ($n = 17$)
- 18 months ($n = 20$)
- 36 months ($n = 9$).

Findings were recorded for the three sample groups prior to and after their participation in the 2-day C&R refresher course.

The complexity of each technique could have some bearing on how much the students retained between and during courses of training. Thus, a rating scale was developed to break down the 'smooth' orthodox competences of the 10 essential techniques into discrete chunks, which would enable observation of the significant parts of the whole. The 'complexity' rating scale was based on how many components there were to the essential technique. For example, technique 1 is rated as 0–4, which meant that there were four parts to the whole movement in which the student should display ability (Table 18.2).

Table 18.2. Complexity of 10 essential care and responsibility techniques

Technique	Movements	Totals
1 Principles of a wrist hold	1 Block 1 Bent wrist 1 Bent arm 1 Pressure if needed	0–4
2 Principles of a straight arm hold	1 Secure below elbow 1 Pressure on elbow or above 1 Direction of the elbow	0–3
3 Securing the head and airway	1 Back of head 1 Front of head 1 Chin 1 Back of head	0–4
4 Transfer of hold – standing	2 Inward rotation 1 Thumb in back of hand 1 Finger/thumb 1 Secure elbow 1 Quarter turn 1 Take through	0–7
5 Transfer of hold – front	1 Resting position 1 Hand position 1 Change grip 1 Move body position 2 Lift arm and extend 1 Quarter turn the knuckles 1 Take through 1 Knees to block 1 Take back to resting position	0–10

Table 18.2. (contd)

Technique	Movements	Totals
6 Transfer of hold – back	1 Resting position	
	1 Hand position	
	1 Elbow between knees	
	1 Forearm parallel with thighs	
	1 Rotate hand	
	1 Secure elbow	
	1 Reposition arm	
	1 Take through	
	1 Finger/thumb	
	1 Block	0–5
7 Removal of hands from object	1 Approach correctly	
	1 Secure elbow	
	1 Secure hand to object	
	2 Apply thumb hold	
	1 Apply principles	0–6
8 Front stranglehold – release	1 Side on	
	1 Arm up	
	1 Walk away	0–3
9 Rear stranglehold – release	1 Maintain airway	
	1 Step behind	
	1 Turn head into body	
	1 Diversion	0–4
10 Hair grabs	1 Secure hand	
	1 Curl wrist	
	1 Pressure elbow	
	1 Move body	0–4

Results

Cohort 1 (updating within 12 months) consisted of 5 female and 12 male ($n = 17$) students; 5 were Ashworth members of staff and 12 were from the NHS. This group experienced a 70% skills diminution within 12 months, although, after update training, 72.3% of the skills had been retained. The majority of students experienced some skills diminution in all techniques, although the diminution did not necessarily relate to the complexity of the techniques as one might have expected. Skill retention was improved after training in all technique areas (Table 18.3). No significant difference between female and male, or Ashworth and non-Ashworth, students was noted by the instructors.

Cohort 2 (updating within 18 months) consisted of 7 female and 13 male ($n = 20$) students; 8 were Ashworth members of staff, and 12 were from the from the NHS. This group experienced a 75% diminution of skills after 18 months; 61.5% of the skills were retained after update training. In all the techniques, the amount of skills diminution was over 66%, with the exception of technique 6 (transfer hold to the back). In every technique, there was an improvement in performance after updating (Table 18.4). No significant difference between female and male, or Ashworth and non-Ashworth, students was noted.

Table 18.3. Cohort 1 findings: update training within 12 months ($n = 17$)

ET	Before updating		After updating	
	SD	SR	SD	SR
1	10	7	7	10
2	11	6	2	15
3	15	2	6	11
4	9	8	3	14
5	13	4	6	11
6	9	8	6	11
7	13	4	7	10
8	13	4	1	16
9	13	4	4	13
10	13	4	5	12
% Skills retained	**70**	**30**	**27.7**	**72.3**

ET = essential technique; SD = skill diminution; SR = skill retention.

Table 18.4. Cohort 2 findings: update training within 18 months ($n = 20$)

ET	Before updating		After updating	
	SD	SR	SD	SR
1	16	4	6	14
2	14	6	6	14
3	16	4	10	10
4	16	4	9	11
5	17	3	10	10
6	12	8	4	16
7	17	3	12	8
8	15	5	8	12
9	14	6	8	12
10	13	7	4	16
% Skills retained	**75**	**25**	**38.5**	**61.5**

ET = essential technique; SD = skill diminution; SR = skill retention.

Cohort 3 (updating within 36 months) consisted of 4 female and 5 male ($n = 9$) students; 5 were Ashworth members of staff, and 4 were from the NHS. This group experienced an 85.6% skills diminution after 3 years and a 52.2% retention of skills after update training. Skills diminution was heaviest in this cohort. Skills retention after updating was improved in every technique except number 7 (removal of hands from object); however, the overall retention rate was disappointing (Table 18.5). No significant difference between female and male, Ashworth and non-Ashworth, students was noted.

Table 18.5. Cohort 3 findings: update training within 36 months ($n = 9$)

ET	Before updating		After updating	
	SD	SR	SD	SR
1	6	3	3	6
2	7	2	1	8
3	9	0	4	5
4	9	0	6	3
5	8	1	4	5
6	7	2	3	6
7	8	1	8	1
8	8	1	6	3
9	7	2	2	7
10	8	1	6	3
% Skills retained	**85.6**	**14.4**	**47.8**	**52.2**

ET = essential technique; SD = skill diminution; SR = skill retention.

Discussion

Figure 18.1 illustrates the percentage of skills retention of the cohorts represented in this survey. Skills diminution is greatest within the first 12 months (a 70% skills loss) of initial training, leakage of skills being more gradual after this time (75% at 18 months, and 85.6% at 36 months). Updating at 12 months also appears to offer optimum results, 72.3% of the skills taught being retained (61.5% at 18 months, and 52.2% at 36 months). These findings support the assertion that a periodic updating or refreshment of skills should be offered 12 months post-initial training. However, the findings raise some scepticism about the assertion that a whole initial course requires repeating if the update does not occur after 12 months (as 30% of the skills are still present at 12 months and 25% at 18 months). This indicates that update courses could be at least 25% shorter than initial courses and that course content needs to be delivered flexibly to assist students to address their skills deficits in the timeframe available for training.

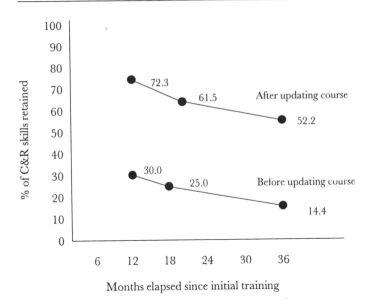

Figure 18.1. Care and responsibility (C & R) skills retention related to periodic updating (%).

This survey was undertaken on a small scale so any generalisation of findings should be made with this in mind. C&R techniques are rapidly evolving; thus, the 'essential techniques' that formed the orthodoxy for this survey will change over time as new techniques are added and others deleted in the search for more effective but less invasive interventions that maximise freedom of choice and dignity for the patient. It is pleasing to note that the scandalous phrase (not uncommon in the late 1980s) 'the therapeutic use of pain' is no longer heard – an indication of the way in which things have progressed.

It is not known whether there are more incidents requiring the use of C&R in high-security hospitals when compared with the NHS. If C&R is used less in the NHS, it may be that Ashworth staff retain more of their competences because of more frequent practice or opportunities for training. However, no major differences between Ashworth and non-Ashworth students (in terms of the assimilation rate of psychomotor skills) was noted. More work is needed in this area.

Skill diminution on entry to courses becomes more marked as the interval between training and updating increases, and the ability to refresh skills seems to be less pronounced as the interval between training grows. The ability to refresh skills may be affected by the individual's learning style, although it is also possible that the teaching techniques in use may be subjected to experimentation and improvement. Indeed, more efficient forms of training might enable shorter courses to be offered, which would assist in the release of staff. More effective forms of teaching might help to reduce the fatigue that some students feel in their upper limbs at the end of a course. This survey suggests that a longitudinal study of C&R training frequency, teaching techniques and individual learning styles is warranted.

The Health and Safety at Work Act 1974 created a statutory imperative related to the reasonable provision of training for staff, and Department of Health and Social Security circular HE(76)11 (1976) placed an onus upon employers to provide guidance to their staff regarding the management of violent/potentially violent situations. Ashworth honoured these requirements and, in so doing, set an arbitrary baseline for training in the management of physical confrontation as 2 days per annum for front-line nurses, to be undertaken within 12 months of the initial training. This was based upon received wisdom.

This survey demonstrated that the '12-month rule' should be followed as C&R skills are noticeably diminished after 12 months without training. It also showed that the ability to relearn techniques is affected by the time interval between updates.

Conclusions

Based upon the outcomes of the survey, the recommendation that staff members should receive annual updating in C&R skills training was affirmed. It was also suggested that experimentation should occur with teaching techniques to see whether more effective forms of delivery could be identified that might enhance skills retention in students (whilst being mindful of issues of individual learning style and the ability to participate in interpersonal training events). It was recommended that a further study, over a longer period and using predominantly Ashworth staff as the sample, should be undertaken by the C&R team.

References

Aiken F, Tarbuck P (1995) Practical ethical and legal aspects of care of the assaultive individual. In Kidd B, Stark C (Eds) Care of the Aggressive Individual. London: Gaskell.

Bates A, McCourt M, Tarbuck P (1997) Care of the Aggressive Individual. London: Royal College of Nursing.

Dale C, Rae M, Tarbuck P (1995) Changing the culture in a special hospital. Nursing Times 91(30): 33–5.

Department of Health and Social Security (1976) Management of the Violent/Potentially Violent Individual. Circular 76(11). London: DHSS.

Epsilon Publishers (1994) Practical Aspects of Managing Violence. Open Learning Modules 1, 2 and 3. London: Epsilon.

Kidd B, Stark C (Eds) (1995) Care of the Aggressive Individual. London: Gaskell.

Parkes P (1996) Control and restraint training: a study of its effectiveness in a medium secure psychiatric unit. Journal of Forensic Psychiatry 7(3): 525–34.

Ritchie J (1984) The Death of Michael Martin at Broadmoor Hospital (The Ritchie Report). Unpublished report by Julie Ritchie QC. Broadmoor Hospital, London

Royal College of Nursing (1992) Seclusion, Control and Restraint. London: Royal College of Nursing.

Royal College of Nursing (1994) Syllabus of Training for Instructors of Control and Restraint. London: Royal College of Nursing.

St John Ambulance (1992) First Aid Manual, 5th Edn. London: St John Ambulance Brigade.

Stansfield R (1998) Control and Restraint Training. Unpublished thesis, University of Salford, Salford.

Tarbuck P (1992a) Ethical standards and human rights. Nursing Standard 7(6): 27–30.

Tarbuck P (1992b) Use and abuse of control and restraint. Nursing Standard 6(52): 30–2.

Tarbuck P (1994) PREP in action: the Ashworth model. Professional Update 2(7): 52–3.

Index